THE
GOOD BOOB
BIBLE

Dai Davies – to my dear wife Julie
Miles Berry – to my darling Fiona for being able
to see the good and inspiring me to be better.
To Alexandra for inspiring wonder at her being.

Both authors wish to acknowledge the thousands of patients that have allowed us to indulge our passion for the art of surgery. We also recognise the debt to the countless surgeons who have inspired and instructed us in the science of surgery.

A special thank you goes to Carla Gilbey for her diplomatic and organisational efforts in channelling the authors' enthusiasm into this comprehensible and readable manuscript.

THE
GOOD BOOB
BIBLE

Your complete guide to breast augmentation surgery

**Miles G Berry MS, FRCS (Plast),
Dai Davies FRCS**

with Maxine Heasman

JOHN BLAKE

Published by Metro Publishing
an imprint of John Blake Publishing Ltd
3 Bramber Court, 2 Bramber Road,
London W14 9PB, England

www.johnblakepublishing.co.uk

www.facebook.com/Johnblakepub   facebook

twitter.com/johnblakepub   twitter

First published in paperback in 2013

ISBN: 978-1-78219-019-6

British Library Cataloguing-in-Publication Data:

A catalogue record for this book is available from the British Library.

Design by www.envydesign.co.uk

Printed in Great Britain by CPI Group (UK) Ltd

1 3 5 7 9 10 8 6 4 2

Papers used by John Blake Publishing are natural, recyclable products made
from wood grown in sustainable forests. The manufacturing processes
conform to the environmental regulations of the country of origin.

Every attempt has been made to contact the relevant copyright-holders,
but some were unobtainable. We would be grateful if the
appropriate people could contact us.

CONTENTS

PREFACE

THE ULTIMATE
BREAST

'The Germans treated their women with esteem and confidence; I consulted them on every occasion of importance and fondly believe that in their breasts resided a sanctity and wisdom more than human.'

The Middle Ages, The Witch, The Virgin, and the Chatelaine: A Short History of Women John Langdon-Davies, 1938

FOREWORD

KNOWLEDGE IS POWER

B reast augmentation (BA) remains the most common cosmetic surgery operation on both sides of the Atlantic (*see* Figs. 1 and 2) and continues to rise in popularity. Advances and improvements in both the implants available and the techniques possible make the procedure more reliable. As expectations continue to rise, it is vital that the individual has a realistic idea of the outcome based on her own unique tissues.

Informed decision-making gives the best possible chance of optimal result and patient satisfaction and requires clear communication of the risks and benefits. On the one hand we have the internet, media and friends that bombard us all with far too much information.

Conversely, the majority of women considering breast augmentation have no medical training to put the surgical issues into context.

While modern anaesthesia is immensely safe, there are still potential side effects or complications that must be weighed up, i.e. pros and con as well as trade-offs when making a decision. No single operation fits all.

Breast enhancement is real surgery; it has lifelong consequences and will probably require some maintenance surgery in the future.

Due to the fact that a consultation allows limited time for the surgeon to impart their wealth of information and experience, the authors (two breast-specialist cosmetic surgeons) were encouraged to write this book in combination with contributions from two women who have themselves undergone BA, the idea being to bring together the relevant aspects of breast augmentation in an informative, readable and current source of reference for prospective patients. We hope our aim of being comprehensive yet clear has been achieved and have provided some scientific background and suggested further reading for those who wish to delve deeper.

Happy reading and remember, knowledge is power. Best of luck!

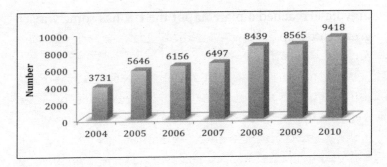

Fig. 1: Annual figures for BA performed in the UK over the last five years. Note these figures are those collated by The British Association of Aesthetic Plastic Surgeons (BAAPS), which records numbers only for its members; around 20,000 are believed to be performed annually by all providers.

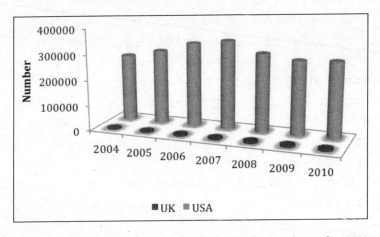

Fig. 2: The same figures for BA performed in the UK compared with those of the USA. The American figures

may have reached a plateau but the UK has some way to go to catch up

1

INTRODUCTION:
WHY DO WOMEN HAVE THEIR BREASTS ENLARGED?

MAXINE HEASMAN, AUTHOR OF *THE ULTIMATE CLEAVAGE*, GIVES A PERSONAL ACCOUNT.

Ever since my late teens I had been unhappy with the size of my breasts. Even though back then I considered them too small, they were very firm and pert so I could not really complain too much. I never regularly wore bras as I had nothing much to fill the cups; there would always be a dimple in the bra material due to the lack of substance behind it! This lack of support over the years meant my 34A breasts inevitably gave way to gravity. The final straw came when I saw myself topless on the beach on a holiday video. I looked awful! What little I had looked all droopy and saggy; I realised my breasts were past their peak and would never be the same again. It was then that I knew there

1

was nothing else for it: I had to have my breasts improved with implants.

I was worried and confused about so many things and absolutely petrified of going under the anaesthetic. How I wished then that I could speak to someone about my concerns, not a surgeon or a clinic but someone who had been through it herself and would really know what I was experiencing. I know it sounds corny, but I started looking at modern female celebrities and decided if they could go through with it and come out looking as wonderful as they do, then so could I. It is fair to say that every celebrity with breast implants was an inspiration to me.

Eventually, after many months of dithering and pondering I made my decision and I will never look back. My new figure has given me so much more confidence and a completely new outlook on life. I now walk into a lingerie department and know that I can wear almost anything in stock and look sexy in it. In the days of my 34A all I could do was look with envy at the sexy bras, knowing full well that if I tried to wear them I would look ridiculous rather than sexy.

MOTIVATION

For most women, breasts symbolise femininity and consequently, having small ones can lead to a feeling of being unfeminine. If you do not feel feminine, you do not feel sexy and these two aspects alone can lead to feelings of insecurity and inferiority. Many women do not let their partners see them naked for months, sometimes years, due to unhappiness with the way they look. If a woman's small breasts are really causing her concern, it seems as if they are glaringly obvious to everyone else – it's as if she has a big red spot on the end of her nose and there's a tendency to assume everyone is looking at it. In reality, most people will look at the woman as a whole and probably not even think twice about the size of her breasts. Of course, there will always be men who will talk to a woman's breasts instead of her face, but that's an exception!

There will not be a day that goes by without seeing curvy full-breasted women in advertising, magazines or films, however, and it is this continual image portrayed by the media that can exaggerate feelings of unhappiness with their breasts in women. Some live with this self-consciousness but others may decide to opt for cosmetic surgery.

This unhappiness can result from:

- A failure of normal breast development at puberty, resulting in small breasts or breasts that differ in size and/or shape.
- Beautiful breasts before or during pregnancy, which are lost after breastfeeding.
- An improvement for other personal reasons.

'I never developed much to begin with...'
Inadequate breast development during puberty

produces breasts that do not appear normal. An abnormal shape may be either a deformity or an imbalance with the rest of a woman's figure. If the breasts develop abnormally during puberty, their shape can be abnormal and can affect how she feels about herself. *No woman has two breasts exactly the same* and sometimes the amount of variation in breast shape and size is large. Imagine the difficulty in trying to buy clothing, dressing to feel normal and how you might feel when clothing is removed.

'I lost everything I had after my baby...'

After pregnancy, the breasts will have been stretched and there is an enlarged skin envelope, with less breast tissue to fill it. The result is an empty upper breast and a droopy appearance of the lower breast.

'I want to improve for personal reasons...'

The third group of women who seek augmentation usually wish to improve the shape and/or size of the breast for a variety of personal reasons. These are women who want to feel better, to be the best they can be. The reasons are personal and every woman has the right to optimise any aspect of her appearance.

'Wanting to be normal...'

There is nothing wrong with wanting to feel normal and to be the best you can be. We all have an idea of normality created by media, including magazine advertising.

WHAT *IS* NORMAL?

If you ask 100 women, you might get 100 different answers. What is normal is personal to each individual and important to you alone. Wanting to feel normal and to be the best you can be are human traits that motivate and reward on a personal level.

Women's breasts are special to them, special in ways that may differ among women and special to each woman in a personal way. Breasts change significantly during a lifetime. Ageing alters the shape and position of a woman's breasts and is not necessarily consistent; they are also never the same.

As a result of this constant change, a woman may view her breasts differently at different times. The best breast at one time may not necessarily be so at another.

EXPECTATIONS: WILL I BE HAPPY?

The best breast is the natural female breast until nature misses a beat, takes its toll or a woman decides her breasts are not how she would like them to be. Although it sounds obvious, the only truly natural breast is a completely natural one. An augmented breast is not totally natural and you should not expect it to be. However, a well-performed augmentation should leave you with a better shape than you had pre-op.

If you want totally natural breasts, you should probably not have breast augmentation (BA)! On the other hand, if the benefits outweigh the trade-off and the risks of BA are acceptable to you, augmentation provides options that can improve what you cannot improve or restore.

Your expectations for augmentation must be realistic for you to be happy with the results. The goal of augmentation is to improve the size and shape of the breasts to the extent that the results meet your goals and you can have a more positive self-image. Although these feelings may allow you to project a more open, positive image to others, the only completely predictable change is larger breasts.

This is an operation on the breasts, not the brain!

Positive psychological effects are common and widely reported, but not necessarily predictable. Certainly, your breast augmentation cannot be expected to have any predictable effect on other people. Some will notice and others may not, depending on your choice of clothing and breast exposure. Your love life and relationship may improve, or it may not. The breasts are only one of many factors that affect the quality of one's love life. A better figure does not necessarily guarantee more modelling jobs or an actress more roles. The decision to have a breast augmentation must be based on realistic personal objectives that you should discuss with your surgeon.

CONCLUSION

There are many women who will be quick to comment that we should be happy with what we have been given and not try to change ourselves. This book makes no such judgements: it has been written for those who do wish to change the way they look. It will, however, bring to your attention many aspects of the procedure that require careful consideration, balancing compromises and trade-offs.

A FEW COMMENTS FROM PATIENTS

'I have been flat-chested all my life and teased because of it. My ex-husband used to be cruel to me and call me half a woman. My present partner never mentions my chest.'

'I have always wanted bigger boobs. I have lost a lot a lot of weight and my boobs have got even smaller; a 36A is too small now. Well, it was my 50th birthday in June 2011 and my husband said if I wanted them done, he will pay for them as a 50th birthday present.'

'My partner helped me to save some of the cost, but I had to borrow the remainder from my bank although I did not think they would approve of me spending money on cosmetic surgery so I made out that I wanted to buy a car!'

'I never let him see me full frontal; I keep myself covered up. My two teenage daughters are very voluptuous and this makes me feel even more inferior – I just want a nice bust to feel like a normal person for once in my life.'

'My feelings go back to being nineteen years of age when I was as thin as a poker. I eventually developed and was quite content with myself, but two of my friends (who were all large-breasted) used to rib me. I did not think at that time that they were all a lot fatter than me and most of it was probably fat anyway. If I am perfectly honest I remember even writing to an agony aunt, who more or less told me to be happy with the rest of my life. My partner's previous wife was built like Pamela Anderson and I think that sometimes he may compare me with her. I tell myself that I have a better personality to compensate! The bottom line is I have other problems, i.e. stretch marks, broken veins in my legs, and all the signs of maturity. I can live with them, cover them up, anything, but this is a real deep problem, which has taken away my self-confidence.'

'The thought of having bigger, firmer, and shapely boobs occupies almost every thought. I have wanted implants since the birth of my third child, six years ago. They have become less firm, and now they look like two wet socks dangling on a washing line. I look like I have an old women's chest now; my nipples point outwards and what I have got flops about, and I am feeling totally miserable.'

'I am only 34AA and I feel really unfeminine; it really does get me down and depressed. I would be so happy with the B cup.'

'I was constantly subjected to cruel jokes about my bust by boys and girls alike. I wore padded bras, even under my halter-neck tops. I am sick of being called a little girl. Although I like to wear sexy clothes, I do not feel womanly ever.'

'I get really depressed at the moment because I feel like I have a little girl's figure. I have even split with my husband over it through jealousy – I do not like him looking at other women, even my own sister (who, I might add, has quite a bit up top). I have had both my sister and her husband take the mickey out of me and made me cry many a time. I do not even go to family parties because I am not happy with myself – I have let it rule my life quite a bit.'

IF YOU DON'T KNOW WHERE YOU'RE GOING, YOU ARE UNLIKELY TO GET THERE!

Let us start by assuming you would like to have breasts that are beautiful, or at least better than they are now.

- What is a beautiful breast?
- What is better than they are now?

The more clearly you define your expectations and the better you communicate individual and specific desires to your surgeon, the more likely you will achieve your goals.

A good place to start is to make a list: What do you dislike about your breasts? Here are some examples.
- My breasts are too small for my figure
- I wish the top of me matched the bottom
- I cannot fill up any bra
- I wish I could wear a T-shirt or top without a bra
- I am sick and tired of buying things to fit the bottom and having to spend more money altering or filling the top
- 'Cleavage' is not a word in my vocabulary
- Every bathing suit I buy must contain helpful devices
- My upper breasts look like ski slopes – no, they look worse than a ski slope!
- I wish I had what I had before I was pregnant *or* I wish I had what I had when I *was* pregnant.

What would you like? List the basics based on what you know and refine your list after reading this book. For example:
- Fuller upper breasts
- More cleavage

- A certain bra 'cup' size
- Bulkier breasts, not huge but proportionate to my figure
- Larger natural breasts
- A better shape to my breasts
- Please fix my weird nipples
- More equal in size and shape
- 'Jordan' or 'Beckham' breasts – large, round and globular.

Now study your list carefully and ask yourself if, in the long term, you are willing to live with your choices.

THE BOTTOM LINE

Do not let window-shopping of pictures in magazines or surgeons' boasting books or the internet fool you about reality. Consider *your own* tissues!

2

THE ORIGIN AND DEVELOPMENT OF THE BREAST

The word 'mammal' derives from the Latin *mammalis*, meaning 'of the breast', indicating that mammals conceive and develop their young within the uterus and after birth, nourish them with milk produced by the mammary glands. Any word containing 'mamma' or 'mammo' therefore refers to the breast – for example, 'mammoplasty' indicating plastic surgery of the breast.

EMBRYOLOGY

As with teeth and feathers, breasts develop from between the two layers of embryonic skin, and are, in fact, modified sweat glands. Both men and women develop breasts from the same embryological tissue. The milk lines are two vertical lines formed by thickenings of the epidermis (skin) called the mammary ridges and these are along the underside of mammals of both sexes. They extend from the armpit to the groin and develop in the embryo. This milk line fragments into individual buds, which in primates develop only in the chest area whereas in other animals, such as in pigs and dogs, they develop along the entire length of the trunk.

Nipples can develop anywhere along the milk line. Most humans have two nipples, but in some cases extra or accessory nipples will develop along the milk line. Sometimes women can grow extra breasts (e.g. in the armpit), but this is very rare.

In pious early Christian times, extra nipples or breast tissue were associated with witchcraft. Hence, witch hunters were allowed to inspect women and those found to have any extra nipples were sentenced to death by burning. More modern reference to the stigma of extra nipple(s) can be found in Ian Fleming's *The Man With the Golden Gun*, where Scaramanga plays the James Bond baddie.

ANTHROPOLOGY

Because primates live in trees and have to carry their offspring around with them, a small litter of one allows much more freedom for climbing. Primates have therefore evolved over time to produce a single child with each pregnancy, thus only one pair of breasts.

All primates, except the human female, have flat chests when not lactating.

Primates usually walk on all fours, which has the effect of concealing the chest. Sexual signals are therefore displayed from behind through the rump and are a key mating stimulus. A human female stands upright and so her breasts are the primary sexual signal, while the buttocks are relatively flat and concealed.

The anthropologist, Desmond Morris, conjectured that the breasts mimic the buttocks as one of the prime areas of sexual signal transmission and their success in this regard has interfered with their primary physical function, that of producing milk. The obvious and clearly displayed primate rump plays a significant role in mating signals because primates walk on all fours. This is completely opposite in the human as we stand upright on two legs, so the female breasts are a significant feature in display. Often the cleavage mimics the buttocks.

BREAST DEVELOPMENT

The breast bud present at birth is sensitive to the mother's hormones; in particular prolactin and oxytocin, which can occasionally stimulate milk production from the newborn breast, the so-called 'Witch's Milk'.

In the human at puberty the breast bud responds to the female hormone, oestrogen, increasing the volume of breast tissue and thereby creating the adult breast. This is highly variable between women and even those closely related, such as mothers, daughters and sisters.

Occasionally, the breasts are very sensitive to oestrogen and it is possible to develop giant breasts, so-called 'Virginal Hyperplasia' or 'Gigantomastia', resulting in breasts weighing as much as 7–8kg (15–17lb), with the nipple hanging down well below the navel.

At puberty, it is not unusual for the male breast to go through a hormonal change, which if marked results in a condition called Gynaecomastia but this often resolves itself with time. It is said that one in ten males develop Gynaecomastia, be it from excess breast tissue or fat, but only a few patients request surgery.

Obesity and the greater use of oestrogenic hormones in the food chain may be behind the greater prevalence seen these days, including former prime ministers and pop moguls alike. In the UK, male breasts (so-called 'moobs') provided the fastest-growing cosmetic surgery procedure in 2010.

The areola of the breast is virgin pink at puberty. With pregnancy it changes in colour, becoming darker, and also enlarges. The areola also has modified sweat glands, which increase in size with pregnancy and are called 'Montgomery's tubercles'. These glands produce a fatty secretion, which is believed to provide biological skincare to the area during breastfeeding. The secretions are also thought to transmit sexual signals through their odour, known as pheromones.

SIZE

The size of the adult female breast is determined by:
- Genetics – smaller-breasted mothers tend to have daughters with smaller breasts
- Breast bud sensitivity to oestrogen
- Degree of obesity – thinner women generally have smaller breasts.

The breast itself consists of glandular tissue, which makes and secretes milk, with the rest being fat. In the non-lactating breast the ratio of fat to breast tissue is approximately 1:1, increasing to 1:2 as the breast gears up for milk production and breastfeeding. Naturally, these proportions vary with the overall size and obesity (i.e. fat content) of the subject. The breast tissue itself lies centred behind the nipple-areola complex (NAC), with the fat mostly located around the edges of the breast.

With pregnancy, the breasts increase in volume and also during breastfeeding. This is in part due to an increase in the amount of glandular tissue and an increased blood supply. It is therefore important when undergoing cosmetic surgery that the mother is no longer breastfeeding. Usually it is advised that a minimum period of three months is allowed between cessation of breastfeeding and any cosmetic surgery.

Female breasts also vary in size with weight gain and loss, the menstrual cycle and the contraceptive pill.

SYMMETRY

Breast development is also subject to a degree of variability between the two sides and few women have identical breasts. On occasion there is a marked difference in size between the two sides that is known as asymmetry.

While this can improve with time, scientific studies show that up to 80 per cent of mature women have asymmetric breasts – in size or shape, or even both. At the extremes of development a woman may have one normal sized breast and have failed to develop on the other side (Breast Hypoplasia or Aplasia).

BREAST FUNCTION

In humans, the breast has two functions: nurture (for milk production) and sexual.

Milk production (nurture)

Usually, there are between 4–18 lactiferous ducts, which take the milk from the breast's glandular tissue to the nipple. When a baby feeds on the breast, it actually takes into its mouth both the nipple and the areola and squeezes by holding, with its gums squirting the milk out and sucking at the same time. In monkeys, the nipple is longer and therefore breastfeeding is easier, so the breasts can be smaller. The first milk that is taken is called 'colostrum' and is very important because it contains antibodies to many of the more common infections absorbed by the just-born baby, providing it with initial protection.

The overall shape of the breast is like an orb. Firstly, to decrease heat loss as relatively high temperatures are required for milk production. Another reason is that the human baby has a very small lower jaw compared to that of primates. If the breast is too flat, it cannot breathe when suckling.

Sexual

Women regard their breasts as important secondary sex characteristics with a fundamental role in sexual attractiveness. They identify a great deal of their femininity and sense of self-appreciation with their breasts; not only the size and shape but also the way they feel. The breasts in this sexual role are also importantly tactile. During arousal the nipple becomes erect and the breasts can increase in size by up to 25 per cent. Both the nipples and the breast skin become more sensitive and some women can develop a red, measles-like blush before orgasm.

CULTURAL SIGNIFICANCE

The breast has occupied a multitude of different vogues and roles throughout the ages. For example, its central importance in nourishment is underscored by the multi-breasted Mother Earth goddess, Cybele, worshipped since Neolithic times. The 'Venus de Milo' captures the tail end of Greek civilisation and is still held to epitomise an optimal female form.

History also has it that certain warrior women in antiquity from central Turkey were known as Amazons. They had one of their breasts amputated to allow them to use a bow and arrow with greater efficiency. This has led to the term 'amazia' – used to describe those who develop only one breast. The Greco-Roman ideal female was often rather masculine, with an emphasis on the muscularity of the body with relatively small breasts.

The mood of society has also proven highly influential in the representation of the female breast. For instance during the Middle Ages with the Church's puritanical outlook, breasts were disguised and made to look as small as possible. They did, however, link the fundamental nutritional aspect directly to spirituality and might be considered the original pin-ups. The explosive creativity of the Renaissance saw breasts being depicted much larger.

While the voluptuousness of the abdomen previously held sway, the sensual focus returned to the cleavage – so much so that Louis XIV demanded lower necklines as a sign of devotion to both him and God.

War and liberation have claimed the breast and were adopted by the French Republic. The symbolic Marianne, with breast bared, leads her people out of the revolution and into a new future, promising freedom, equality and brotherhood.

Of course we all know that 'sex sells', but the connection between tyres and breasts is tenuous at best. Pirelli's now-iconic calendar has, however, subverted the establishment: originally a product designed to age away on the walls of a mechanic's garage, these calendars now not only attract the cream of the photographic world but big-name models, too.

CLEAVAGE

Many women are also concerned about their cleavage and some regard it as a tool for flirting or seduction. Strictly speaking, the cleavage is the space between the breasts that overlies the breastbone. It is thought by some to mimic the cleavage between the buttocks – this depends on both breast shape and volume and to a lesser extent, the underlying chest wall. Modern-day bras and corsets – and of course surgery – have fulfilled the expectations of fashion by changing the shape, size and position of the female breast.

Sometimes there is little or no cleavage and one breast merges into the other – 'symmastia'. Although the condition can occur naturally, it may also be a consequence of poorly performed breast augmentation, whereby pocket dissection has been excessive or too large an implant has led to gradual tearing of the middle fibres over the breastbone. Also known as 'uniboob' or 'bread-loaf breast', in the most extreme cases the two implants actually come to touch each other. Correction requires surgery, reduction of implant volume and is technically difficult, with results not guaranteed.

THE CHANGING BREAST

As detailed in the next chapter (The Anatomy of the Breast, page 26), the breast has several supporting structures, including the inframammary fold (IMF) and Cooper's ligaments. Unfortunately, with age, pregnancy and excessive weight gain, these stretch and the breast droops. With time, the breast becomes supported less and less by the ligaments and IMF, and increasingly by the chest wall.

The breasts are never static in size and shape and consistency. Here, Shakespeare's *The Seven Ages of Man* has been paraphrased to describe the changing female breast:
- The nipple breast of childhood
- The breast bud of puberty
- The pointed breast of adolescence
- The firm breast of the young adult. It is said that the physical peak is achieved around the age of twenty-five
- The full breast of motherhood and droopiness (ptosis) starts
- The sagging breast of middle age
- The pendulous breast of old age.

THE ORIGIN AND DEVELOPMENT OF THE BREAST

The depiction of breasts makes it easy for the artist to change their size and shape, though not the photographer. In general, the photographer tries to show maximum protrusion of the breast with minimal droop and therefore there is only a short phase of a woman's life, in her late teens and early twenties, when her breasts are at their biological and photogenic peak. This explains why the *Sun* newspaper's Page 3 girls all fall into a fairly narrow age range, with a tendency to rapid replacement by younger models.

3

THE ANATOMY OF THE BREAST

Breasts are highly variable in size, shape and colour. Anatomically speaking, they are rounded organs comprising glandular tissue; fat and skin that sit on top of the pectoralis major muscles of the upper chest. Women tend to assess their breasts by either volume (the bra cup size) or cleavage. Surgeons consider the female breast by way of its component parts, which include the base, the mound, the skin envelope and the nipple-areola complex (NAC). It is said that the mean breast weight is 0.5kg (1.1lb) and contributes around 1 per cent to total body weight, although this is highly variable.

ANATOMY OF THE FEMALE BREAST

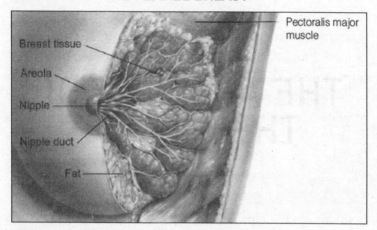

Base

The base of the breast, or footprint, defines the extent of the breast. Highly variable in width, it extends vertically from the second to the sixth ribs. There is a smooth, indistinct take-off at the top, but a well-demarcated crease at the bottom that is very important for supporting the breast and is known as the inframammary fold (IMF). (*see* Fig.3)

The width of the breast is also highly variable and starts at least 1cm (½in) from the midline. At this point the skin is thick and firmly adherent to the breastbone. The breast is always fuller on the outside and larger breasts will protrude more. We all know that breasts tend to move sideways when lying down and this is partly because of the weight but also due to the outwards sloping nature of the chest wall.

The base width is of fundamental importance in determining the optimum implant volume for each woman individually and that's why your surgeon will not be particularly interested in your friend's size of implants unless you share identical chests, preoperative breast volumes and tissue characteristics, to say nothing of height, weight and general body shape.

Mound

The most variable part of the breast, the mound depends on base width, general size and degree of obesity. This is the element that most women seek to improve through breast augmentation, be it for small breasts (hypomastia) or those empty following breast-feeding (post-partum).

In some women the breast has a lateral extension, which extends from the outside towards the armpit. This is known as the 'axillary tail' and can enlarge with pregnancy, resulting in swelling in the armpit. This is not dangerous.

The Inframammary Fold (IMF)

The IMF is an important support structure at the base of the breast. It has been shown to have a slightly different type of connective tissue, in a condensed fashion to hold up the base of the breast. Over time, it descends but is assisted by the shape of the chest; it can be disturbed by poorly performed surgery too.

The skin and soft tissue envelope

Overlying the substance of the gland is what is referred to as the 'envelope'. It comprises skin and subcutaneous tissue and may be tight or loose, according to its relationship with the underlying glandular tissue. When the envelope is loose, the breast droops. This is most frequently seen after pregnancy and breastfeeding or weight loss.

Skin tone and appearance are very important. At puberty the normal skin is thick, with good elastic tone and no stretch marks. The skin is well supported by the underlying fat and breast tissue. With pregnancy or excess weight gain, it becomes thinner and stretches with poor tone. As skin ages it progressively loses the ability to return to normal after being expanded or stretched; stretch marks are permanent reminders of excess force that has strained the skin beyond its natural elastic ability.

It is important to appreciate that the skin and breast tissue together provide the soft tissue that is available to cover a breast implant. Most women have seen the infamous pictures of very skinny celebrities where the prosthesis is visible through the skin.

One of the most important steps in preoperative assessment is evaluation of the soft-tissue available to cover any implant and a caliper is used for the pinch test in order to determine which pocket is best for each individual case.

Shape

The shape is also variable; classically the breast is round or orb-shaped. Shapes vary enormously, with a not uncommon variation being a contracted (smaller) base with a protruding, floppy areola, known as a 'tubular breast' (*see* Fig.4). A surprisingly high proportion of women have some degree of this developmental anomaly and are often somewhat relieved to learn that they are not alone.

Nipple-Areola Complex (NAC)

The NAC, with its central protruding nipple, is surrounded by an area of variably pigmented skin and plays an important role in the apparent age of a breast. When youthful, it sits in the centre of a circular mound. With advancing age, the mound becomes less circular, wider, and the NAC starts to descend.

NAC position relative to the inframammary fold (IMF) is a key defining feature of the breast and the NAC should lie above the IMF. Surgeons have a grading system for the degree of droop (ptosis) that helps to define and plan surgery (*see* Fig.5). Grade I is the mildest, with III being the most severe, where the nipple has descended to lie both below the IMF and at the lowest point of the breast.

When the nipple-areola complex lies below the inframammary groove, a mastopexy or 'hitch up' may be required, as well as breast augmentation (*see also* Chapter 12).

Inverted nipples

Projection of the nipple can vary greatly. If the lactiferous duct is short, it pulls the nipple inwards so that the nipple does not protrude but is drawn into the breast.

There are three grades of inverted nipples, defined by how easily the nipple may be pulled out (protracted) and the degree of fibrosis/length discrepancy of the lactiferous ducts. The condition is important for both aesthetic and functional reasons as severe inversion may prevent breastfeeding.

- Grade I: a nipple that is easily and fully protracted with finger pressure around the areola. It maintains its projection, rarely retracts and is associated with little or no duct deficiency or fibrosis. Also, Grade I inverted nipples may pop up without manipulation or pressure and are alternatively known as 'shy nipples'.
- Grade II: a nipple that can be pulled out, though not as easily as Grade I, but retracts after pressure is released. Breastfeeding may be possible, but is more likely to be very difficult or even impossible. There is a moderate degree of fibrosis and mild retraction of lactiferous ducts. Grade II is the most common form.

- Grade III: describes a nipple that can rarely be physically pulled out and requires surgery to be protracted. Milk ducts are usually constricted and breastfeeding is impossible. Women with Grade III nipple inversion may also experience infections and rashes and struggle with nipple hygiene. Fibrosis is marked and the lactiferous ducts are short.

- There are several operations that can generally be performed under local anaesthesia as a day case to correct this 'abnormality' but all will result in an inability to breastfeed as the ducts are divided.

SUPPORT OF THE BREASTS

As the breasts are subject to the forces of gravity, which pull them down when standing and outwards when lying, they require some natural support in the form of:

- The skin
- Cooper's ligaments
- The chest wall muscles
- The inframammary fold (IMF)
- Chest shape.

Skin

The supportive ability of the skin depends on many factors, including genetic predisposition, age, sun

31

damage, smoking and the breast weight that determines the degree of stretch.

Cooper's ligaments

Cooper's ligaments (as described by the famous 19th-century surgeon, Sir Astley Cooper) extend from the collarbone, much like a curtain, through and around the breast tissue to the IMF. They are important for suspending the breasts but as all women come to know, they stretch with time so allowing sag to develop. This tends to exacerbate loss of fullness in the upper half of the breast.

Chest wall muscles

Not strictly part of the breast, but an important structure in augmentation are the muscles on which the breast sits. The main one is the pectoralis major and is easily recognised in athletes as the upper chest muscles, particularly in sprinters. For many years, breast implants were placed between the muscle and the gland (subglandular). This procedure risks implant visibility in thin patients, and this is something clients are increasingly concerned about. In the 1970s, placement under the pectoralis muscle (submuscular) was described and has grown to be a very popular option. Covering the surface of the pectoralis muscle is a layer of fibrous tissue called the clavipectoral fascia, which also helps to support the breast.

Inframammary Fold

The Inframammary Fold (IMF) appears to be a specialised area of fibrous tissue that has been well studied and forms an important role in both defining the inferior border of the breast and supporting the breast from gravitational descent. Although it may move downwards with age and weight gain, surgery is the usual cause of a low IMF, particularly with large implants.

Shape of the chest

Being wider at the top, the male chest is either straight or a little triangular. The larger chest is designed for running and hunting. Conversely, the female chest is narrower and comes to be wider at the bottom as the lower ribs flare out. It is believed that this provides some support to the female breast.

MAIN LANDMARKS OF THE FEMALE BREAST
Blood supply

The blood supply to the breast comes from three main sources:

- The armpit in the upper outer part
- Perforating vessels from the arteries between the ribs
- The internal mammary artery in the cleavage.

A rich and multiple blood supply allows surgeons to safely cut away parts of the breast, particularly in mastopexy, breast reduction and oncoplastic breast surgery (the combination of cancer surgery techniques and aesthetic surgery to give optimal cosmetic outcomes in cases of breast cancer) without threatening the blood supply to the nipple or other areas of the breast.

LYMPHATIC DRAINAGE

Lymphatic drainage passes predominantly to the axilla (armpit), which is why doctors always prod around in the armpit, should an infection or tumours be suspected.

NERVE SUPPLY

Sensation to the breast is obviously important, with two areas to be considered: the nipple-areola complex (NAC) and the rest of the breast, including skin and the deeper breast tissue.

The degree of nipple sensation varies widely and there is a wide spectrum of what is considered normal. In some there is little and it is relatively unimportant. To others it is very important, with some women achieving orgasm through nipple stimulation alone.

Sensation is transmitted by sensory fibres, which originate from nerves running between the underlying ribs. One of the most important is that between the fourth and fifth ribs as it provides most of the sensation to the nipple-areola complex (NAC). Much of it travels along the surface of the pectoralis muscle in the submammary space, causing it to be more at risk of permanent damage in a submammary than a submuscular pocket dissection.

PRINCIPLES OF BEAUTY

The French surgeon, Moufarrège, looked at various ratios and proportions of aesthetically pleasing breasts. With respect to breast height, as long as it is more than twice and less than four times greater than projection, the breast is attractive. It was also found that height and width should be similar, with the best proportion lying between 0.7 and 1.3. In fact, these figures echo Grecian ideals and phi (Φ) has long held a fundamental importance in art, science and beauty. It is believed that ultimate aesthetic attractiveness conforms to this ratio, which mathematically equates to 1.618. Many parts of the human body obey this rule, from fingers to the facial subunits, but one of nature's best examples is the humble snail shell, with each successive spiral increasing by a factor of precisely 1.618.

CHEST WALL SYMMETRY

Underappreciated by the majority and rarely even noticed by many, the chest wall itself can have a major influence on the final result of breast augmentation. As with most other paired structures, perfect symmetry is rare and it is important that your surgeon looks for, and tells you about it before any surgery.

There are two reasons for this: firstly, the use of standard implants may make the difference appear more obvious and should not be blamed. Imagine building a house on uneven ground: you would not be at all surprised if it did not end up crooked, if no allowances were made for differences.

Secondly, in some cases it is possible to use differing size and shape implants in order to improve any inequality present. While impossible to obtain a perfect result (if the Almighty could not get it right, you should not expect your surgeon to!), significant improvements are possible.

Asymmetry is an area where the use of the new technique of 3D imaging is very helpful, both for the patient in terms of appreciating and understanding the starting position because an image is taken of her own chest, and for the surgeon in operative planning. Your surgeon should also be assessing whether the perceived asymmetry is true or apparent. It is true if there is a difference between the two breasts, whatever the position. Apparent can easily be confused and is rather common because often people do not stand straight: the surgeon can confirm this by looking at your spine for signs of twisting and your shoulders for differences in height. Infrequently found in nature, perfect symmetry is highly prized, being associated with beauty and attractiveness.

As with everything there are varying degrees of asymmetry, from the barely noticeable to the complete absence on one side. There is an uncommon condition that may co-exist with breast underdevelopment: Poland's syndrome. It was first described by Alfred Poland in 1841, while he was still a medical student, and comprises varying degrees of developmental lack of the breast, chest wall musculature (pectoralis major) and the upper limb on the same side. It is the extreme end of the spectrum for failed development and people are usually aware of it early in life.

CASE STUDY

HG, a 36-year-old woman, requested breast augmentation to increase the size of her bust from a AA. She has not had any children and medically, she was in excellent health but a noticeable difference in the two sides of her chest wall was noted at initial consultation.

The preoperative photograph showed differences in the two breasts but not as clearly the underlying chest asymmetry obvious in the flesh. As a result, HG underwent 3D imaging, which helped her to understand the issues and simulate the effect of different implant sizes. In fact due to the unusually large difference of the

---

chest wall sides, both a different size and style of implant were used on each side: a 375cc high profile was used on the right and 290cc moderate profile on the left.

4
FINDING A SUITABLE SURGEON

Choosing the right surgeon is your responsibility. It takes time to research and is probably the single most important step towards obtaining the best possible breast augmentation. Finding a suitable surgeon with all the necessary qualifications and experience is absolutely vital. Not only do good surgeons have better results, but fewer complications too.

Firstly, let us clear up some of the confusion that exists about the name or title your surgeon may use. Neither the Royal College of Surgeons nor the General Medical Council (GMC) recognises cosmetic surgery as a separate specialty, so any doctor can call him- or herself a cosmetic surgeon. This seems to be a particular quirk of the UK and can cause much confusion.

Plastic surgeons can be found on the GMC's Specialist Register and no one else may use this title. The word 'plastic' is derived from the Greek word 'plastos', meaning to shape or mould, and was first used with the word 'rhinoplasty', meaning to modify the shape of a nose. As in every field, plastic surgeons may have a particular training and expertise in only one or two areas. This is known as 'super-specialisation' and has evolved to give safer, better and more reliable outcomes for our patients.

Today, in the UK, cosmetic surgery is performed by plastic, cosmetic, ear, nose & throat (ENT), ophthalmic, oncoplastic and general surgeons, dermatologists, general practitioners and even orthopaedic surgeons, so it would be wise to confirm the specific area of your chosen cosmetic surgeon's training, expertise and experience.

'Aesthetic surgeon' is a title used by some and actually means nothing. All surgeons should be aesthetic in their approach to surgery and this includes orthopaedic, gynaecological and even brain surgeons.

THE NORMAL PATHWAY FOR TRAINING A SURGEON IN THE UK

Medical school training at undergraduate level lasts five years. At the end of that time, the doctor will be awarded Bachelor of Medicine and Bachelor of Surgery (MB, BS or BM BCh) degrees. He/she will then undergo two years' supervised medical training in its generality, including different specialties – all in a hospital environment. The two years are called 'SP1' and 'SP2'.

At the end of this period, anyone intending to be a surgeon will have sat and passed the MRCS (Member of the Royal College of Surgeons) examination. This provides an entrance into surgical training and these days, no one can get in without having made the grade.

There is then a very competitive national selection to be accepted for higher surgical training in a specialty. This takes six years in accredited jobs in hospitals throughout the United Kingdom and often abroad. Each year the trainee's record is examined and progress to the next year depends on a satisfactory assessment. Towards the end of the six years, they will prepare for the FRCS (Fellow of the Royal College of Surgeons) specialist examination (usually in plastic, ENT or maxillo-facial surgery or oncology). Ideally, your breast surgeon should be FRCS (Plast).

At the end of six years of satisfactory training and having passed the FRCS (Plast), the surgeon will obtain a Certificate of Surgical Training (CST) and will be placed on the GMC Specialist Register according to their training. Theoretically, a fully qualified plastic surgeon will spend eight or nine years training; once qualified, most surgeons study for longer. Almost all plastic surgeons will also specialise in cosmetic surgery and as part of this super-specialise in, say, breast augmentation (BA) or facial surgery.

The surgeon can now either apply for a consultant post in the National Health Service (NHS), or go directly into private practice. At this stage most surgeons work as a consultant in the NHS and also take their first tentative steps in a cosmetic surgery practice.

THE GENERAL MEDICAL COUNCIL

This body is empowered by the government to register medical practitioners and grant permission to work in the United Kingdom, either as a general practitioner or as a specialist. Unfortunately, the GMC does not supervise what operations a surgeon can undertake nor does it exclude general practitioners or physicians from undertaking surgery. The question you should ask yourself is: would you let an electrician loose on your plumbing, and vice-versa? And would you expect the best possible result?

Two things to bear in mind

Always check that your surgeon is on the GMC Specialist Register, but in particular which register he/she is on. After all, with the greatest respect you do not want an orthopaedic surgeon well trained in knee replacement undertaking your breast augmentation, which is a possibility.

Secondly, those who have trained in Europe have a reciprocal arrangement whereby it is deemed that having had specialist training from their home country, they can go onto the Specialist Register in the United Kingdom. Most people would agree that the specialist training in some countries is not so exacting as in the UK. So many companies claim their surgeons are all on the GMC Specialist Register, but what you should ask is this: where did they train?

Surgeons have to get admitting rights to private hospitals or clinics to undertake surgery. A few surgeons will have their own operating surgery facility in their offices (as in the US) but this, by and large, is limited to just one or two surgeons in the UK, although more and more dermatologists in particular are developing surgical facilities for liposuction and interventional laser treatment in an office setting or medical spa.

All hospitals are regulated by the Care Quality Commission (CQC), which used to be known as the Healthcare Commission. The CQC regularly inspects hospitals and involves auditing the surgeons and anaesthetists working there. A surgeon has to be assessed by the hospital's Medical Advisory Committee and if their training is deemed inappropriate or if reports from colleagues on their performance (particularly in the operating theatre) are inappropriate, admitting rights to that hospital can be removed. To a certain extent this is a safeguard, however hospitals are under increasing financial pressure and may establish block contracts with commercial organisations to undertake their surgery. Part of that contract will involve accepting surgeons who, if not working for that organisation, would not receive admitting rights to that hospital. The fact that a surgeon has admitting rights to several hospitals is no longer a sign that he is a good surgeon.

One other consideration about admitting rights into hospital is to ask the surgeon where they live and where else they have operating rights. You do not want to have a surgeon who spends one-third of the week operating in Ireland or the United States and the rest of the time in London. Obviously, he/she cannot provide the supervised care that you are entitled to.

COLLEGES AND COSMETIC SURGERY ASSOCIATIONS
These organisations include:

The Royal College of Surgeons – This body supervises the examinations, together with the Specialist Advisory Committee (SAC) of surgeons, and is involved in the supervision of training and research. Most British trained surgeons will be fellows of the Royal College of Surgeons.

BAAPS (The British Association of Aesthetic Plastic Surgeons) – The major society in the United Kingdom associated with the training and supervision in cosmetic surgery. Most British plastic surgeons undertaking cosmetic surgery are members of BAAPS.

BAPRAS (The British Association of Plastic, Reconstructive and Aesthetic Surgery) was until recently the British Association of Plastic Surgery (BAPS) and extended its name along the American lines to include the subspecialty of aesthetic surgery in its title. The mother organisation of British plastic surgery, it has its own world-famous journal, the *Journal of Plastic, Reconstructive & Aesthetic Surgery* (JPRAS).

BACS (British Association of Cosmetic Surgeons) grew out of the fact that surgeons who are not on the GMC Specialist Register, working independently or for the major cosmetic surgery clinics, did not fulfil the admission criteria of the British Association of Aesthetic Plastic Surgeons (BAPRAS) and therefore formed their own society.

ISAPS (The International Society of Aesthetic Plastic Surgery) is a worldwide association involved in the training and dissemination of information on cosmetic surgery. It has its own journal and a few British plastic surgeons are members of ISAPS.

A word of advice: do not be flattered by all these acronyms. The major associations for the United Kingdom mainstream are BAAPS and BAPRAS.

THE BOTTOM LINE

The Specialist Register run by the GMC does not ensure that your surgeon is a well-trained cosmetic surgeon nor that he/she has received high-quality training in the United Kingdom.

BREAST ENLARGEMENT ON THE NHS

Some women (very few) are able to qualify for breast enlargement surgery on the National Health Service. At the present time, the control of spending is undertaken by the PCT (Primary Care Trust) and your GP will refer your case to the PCT for extra funding to pay for your operation. The PCT are not financially capable of funding cosmetic surgery and therefore require exceptional circumstances before they will pay for your surgery. Our present financial climate makes this an even less likely option, although some are finding that the NHS will allow for removal of the defective French PIP implants. What they will not do, however, is to allow replacements!

With the chequered history of breast implants after Trilucent and Hydrogels – which were only rushed to the market in the absence of adequate testing because of the anti-silicone lawsuits in America – it was disappointing that 2010 saw a new problem. The potential for profit led the unscrupulous astray in the French company PIP (Poly-Implant Prothese). Weaker shells were used in the manufacture of implants to cut costs. The barrier layer was removed and so gel bleed is more common. Furniture- rather than medical-grade silicone gel also helped PIP's profit margins, but not of course their patients! Although used by many in the late nineties and early noughties, most independent surgeons had stopped using them by 2006 due to the apparently increased rupture rate observed. Unfortunately, these implants had been passed at Europe's highest level of regulation for medical devices, CE (Conformité Européene). Many of the larger cosmetic companies continued using them right up until the ban in April 2010.

CONTACTING SURGEONS DIRECTLY

With the internet, information on both the subject of breast augmentation and on the availability of surgeons undertaking BA is freely available. There is nothing to stop you from contacting surgeons directly by applying on the internet or through associations such as the British Association of Aesthetic Plastic Surgeons (see Useful Contacts, page 235), who will provide a list of BAAPS members, geographically identified. They will also send you some basic information on the surgical procedure.

When dealing with surgeons directly, it is very important that you find out how experienced they are. Who do they work for and what is their relationship with any other organisation? You should find out from them how many breast augmentation operations they perform each week but remember, volume is not necessarily a measure of a good surgeon: maybe he/she is doing ten a day and doing them badly compared to another surgeon who does just two to three procedures a week, but does them well.

It is also essential that you fully understand what is included in the price quoted to you and whether it is all-inclusive. Some surgeons do not provide a total package cost. Instead they will charge separately for various aspects of care and any complications.

PRIVATE CLINIC OR INDIVIDUAL

Formerly doctors and surgeons were prohibited from advertising their services and the way to get round this was for them to work for private clinics, which were free to advertise anywhere. With the internet doctors and surgeons are now freely able to advertise. As a result, marketing has become an important aspect of cosmetic surgery, which is now a business, and most surgeons will have an expensive website; they may well pay for advertising in magazines and will have a public relations (PR) advisor, too. Naturally, all this represents considerable outlay and so some surgeons continue to work for the private clinics that can obviously spend much more on advertising and marketing.

There are also agents who work without their own clinic premises and act on behalf of a surgeon who will use the facilities of a private hospital. These agents say they give independent advice for which you will be charged, but usually they have a line of referral to one or several particular surgeons.

THROUGH A COSMETIC COMPANY

Why do some of the cosmetic clinics use foreign trained cosmetic surgeons, who have not completed any training in the United Kingdom and have not worked in the NHS? The reasons are as follows:
- They will work for much cheaper rates
- They can obtain much cheaper malpractice insurance from their own country
- They will do the operation quickly and you may be unhappy with the result, at which point you will find that the company says all the problems should be referred to the surgeon who undertook your operation and it is to him that you should address your complaint. The problem is that the surgeon may have returned to his/her original country or else-where in Europe.

The advantage for a surgeon working for a clinic or a company is that he/she is able to receive a steady stream of clients while the clinic handles all the advertising administration and finance. If a surgeon uses a clinic to provide him/her with patients, the chances are he/she will be performing many operations on a weekly basis and should be well practised and experienced, but experience shows that many of these surgeons have trained abroad and sometimes have dubious insurance – here today, gone tomorrow. While the clinics may provide the most competitive cost, they achieve this by paying the surgeon and the anaesthetist as little as possible and use the cheapest available prosthesis. This was certainly the case in the recent scandal of the defective PIP breast prosthesis made in France. Although now banned, thousands were inserted in the UK – almost all by cosmetic surgery clinic companies.

It is important not to think of the clinic and the surgeon as necessarily one and the same. The clinic or agent introduces you to a surgeon and usually takes responsibility for all correspondence to do with arranging consultation and surgery dates but may not guarantee the outcome of surgery and in particular, helping you with any complications, especially late ones.

The onus is still very much on you, the patient, to ask the surgeon all the necessary questions in just the same way as if you had approached him/her directly yourself.

Some women experience hard-sell techniques in which they are persuaded to put down a substantial deposit during the initial consultation before even seeing a surgeon. The most common complaint with many private clinics is the lack of contact after surgery. We have received comments on how the care inside the clinic seemed to fade away once all monies had been paid. Look for a clear schedule of aftercare appointments, complete with emergency contact numbers. This should be arranged for all patients, whether surgery is through a clinic or the surgeon.

Competing now in this market are the large hospital groups that own hospitals throughout the UK. They are looking for the so-called 'self-pay' patients, to whom they offer a package deal. Invariably you will find that it is the most junior surgeons on their books who do the surgery as it is carried out at a cut-price surgical fee compared to the more established consultants. You may also find that from one particular hospital within the group to another there is a wide variation in price. One of the other problems is that they as a group will employ many different surgeons to undertake this surgery, sometimes using it as an inducement to try and get the surgeon to bring his other work to the hospital. There is much variation in the way the operations are carried out, and in the audit and outcome of surgery.

REMEMBER THE FOLLOWING...

- Check whether the person with whom you are speaking is medically qualified and not just a sales representative. Just because they are wearing a white coat, do not assume they are from the medical profession!

- Lots of private clinics offer free consultation, but no matter how informative and helpful they may be, it is essential that you have a full consultation with the actual surgeon who will be performing your operation before agreeing to anything.
- Do not pay out any money or commit yourself to anything until you have had time to think about it and shop around. Even the financial services industry has a 'cooling-off' period!
- Ask what aftercare will be provided. How many postoperative consultations will be provided? Will it be down to you to arrange these with the surgeon or will the clinic make the necessary arrangements?

THE BOTTOM LINE

When dealing with clinics or agents, use your knowledge and apply common sense and intuition.

PERSONAL RECOMMENDATION (PROBABLY BEST OF ALL)

Of all the options available personal recommendation is easiest and perhaps the best way to find a good reputable surgeon. What better introduction than via a blow-by-by account from a happy breast implant patient, especially if you have been able to see her breasts and scars and even feel them beforehand? If you know of someone who has undergone breast augmentation, then talk to them about their experience and ask for the name of their surgeon, if they are happy. A lot of women who consider breast enlargement keep an eye out for relevant articles in magazines and on the television, but remember to interpret what you read with your own knowledge. If you are impressed by another woman's story, there is nothing to stop you from writing to her, c/o the magazine. Your local hairdressing or beauty salon may also know of women who have had breast implants, who are happy to share their experiences.

5

THE CONSULTATION

M any companies provide a long consultation with a co-ordinator, followed by a short consultation with the chosen surgeon. Actually, it should be the other way round.

You evaluate the surgeon, and the surgeon evaluates you!

The surgical consultation forms one, if not *the* most important part of the entire process of your breast augmentation and has several distinct, but overlapping phases:
• Clinical Assessment: fit for surgery and motivation
• Physical Assessment and measurements
• Recommendation: Combination of what the patient

desires and what their individual body safely
allows to give the best and most durable
result
- Information gathering by both patient and surgeon
- Sizing.

There is a standard format to all consultations, with a full clinical history at the start. This is followed by clinical examination when key measurements are taken from the patient. Clinical photographs are also obtained and will be of critical importance as neither patient nor surgeon will be able to adequately recall the preoperative situation after surgery.

While it can be done in a few minutes, remember the old saying: 'you get what you pay for'. Five-minute consultations may appear convenient, but do they allow sufficient time for an exchange of information on both sides? At the very least you should expect twenty to thirty minutes of your surgeon's time for a comprehensive consultation.

WHO IS SUITABLE?

Your surgeon will, or should be making an assessment of your physical and psychological status, in addition to your expectations and how reasonable and achievable they are. If medically fit and well, you should be suitable for the anaesthetic. The surgeon will be seeking to establish this as a prime safety issue because cosmetic surgery is undertaken for want rather than need, so the risk-benefit balance is all-important.

MOTIVATION AND EXPECTATIONS

It is extremely important that the surgeon is able to identify those who have totally unrealistic expectations or unusual reasons for surgery. The former comprise those who often bring in pictures of celebrities or friends and request imitation of one particular aspect, despite being entirely different in their own body make-up. The latter group may mistakenly believe that having larger, fuller breasts will help with intimate relationships or possibly even career progression. One group that frequently ends up being dissatisfied are those pushed into it, unwillingly, by their partner. Since you run all the risks and will have to accept any complications and preoperative discomfort, the choice must be yours.

There is a smaller group who have what is known as 'Body Dysmorphic Disorder' (BDD). A good example of this is patients who have many different cosmetic surgery operations from head to toe and are never satisfied with their body image.

AGE

There is no rigid upper limit, but the minimum age for cosmetic surgery is usually eighteen years as the breast has barely finished growing and developing by this age; some surgeons wait even longer. A small minority of patients are considered for surgery at a younger age: those with significant asymmetry, where one breast remains underdeveloped, causing severe emotional and psychological issues.

It is worth repeating that the female breast is an active organ that will continue to change in size, shape and nature with childbirth, breastfeeding and age. Finally, most will understand that just like joint replacements, being man-made prostheses will not last indefinitely, so the younger the patient, the more likely the need for further surgery later on in life.

PARTNERS

While not completely essential, a supportive partner, family or close family member is a welcome sight during consultation for support throughout the consent process and immediate postoperative period. It is particularly important and helpful in the uncommon event that things do not go entirely according to plan and a complication supervenes.

Another key point is that the prospective patient's partner is generally happy with their loved one; they may otherwise feel left out of what is a potentially very important decision. 'Two heads are better than one' is an apt maxim where informed consent occurs: there is so much information that needs to be taken on board that together the two recall more than one alone. It is, of course, important to understand that the final decision rests with the patient herself.

Try to remember that unless the person you happen to know who has had a BA is your identical twin, her shape, style and size of implant are unlikely to precisely match your own highly individual characteristics!

THE SURGEON'S PAGE

Questions your surgeon is, or should be, asking:

- Is this patient medically fit for an operation?
- Is this patient emotionally fit for an operation?
- Does this patient know what she really wants from this operation?
- Are the patient's expectations realistic? If not, can she be educated to accept what is possible and appropriate for her? If not, does she comprehend the risks and possible complications?
- What is her personal level of understanding and need for information, and am I achieving this?
- Is the patient physically appropriate (symmetry, envelope, ptosis)?
- Is the patient taking the responsibility and accountability for choices she may have made in the short and long term with their trade-offs?

EXAMINING AND MEASURING THE PATIENT

Following a general assessment of the size, shape and

symmetry of your body, the surgeon should examine your breasts for lumps or tenderness, including the armpit for any lymph nodes that can be felt, and assess the skin and breast tissue tone. The most important observation he/she should make and comment on is the position of your nipple in relation to the inframammary fold (IMF). If the nipple-areola complex (NAC) lies at, or above the fold, you are suitable for routine breast augmentation.

If your nipple lies below the groove, you may be suitable for biplanar breast augmentation or, in more droopy cases, especially if the skin is lax with poor tone and striae (stretch marks), a mastopexy augment (*see also* Chapter 12) may be the only way of achieving a satisfactory shape.

Your surgeon should record the consultation on a worksheet which contains many measurements and questions that will allow him/her to make an assessment of what you have, what your tissue quality is like and what implant (shape, pocket and size) will give you the best result.

Key breast measurements taken:
- Sternal notch to nipple-areola complex (SNN)
- Nipple-areola complex to inframammary fold (N-IMF)
- Base width (BW) of breast
- Chest girth.

MEASURING THE SIZE OF THE PROSTHESIS

There is an optimum size and shape of prosthesis that fits with your individual tissue characteristics, which your surgeon should recommend. If this differs to what you, the patient, have as an idea of size then there may be a problem.

When a surgeon advises you on a size he/she should start by looking at the base diameter of the prosthesis sitting on your chest. Of course narrower chests allow a smaller diameter base of prosthesis, whereas a wider chest allows a wider implant and the same goes for the height of the chest. Some people have a long chest, others a short chest, so the footprint of the implant is important.

The next variable is the thickness of the breast skin envelope covering the prosthesis. Ideally, the prosthesis should fill the empty or poorly filled envelope. The reason for this is that any undue pressure caused by a larger prosthesis tends to thin the covering tissues in the long-term. This is particularly the case where younger girls wish to have especially large breasts, what may be called 'exotic'. It is all very well and good for a photograph, but three things will happen:

- Tissues will become thin, thus making any form of reconstruction once the glamour of having large breasts has passed more difficult. The operation of mastopexy with very thin tissues makes moving the nipple upwards precarious.

- The larger the prosthesis, even if placed underneath the muscle, inevitably will drop in time.
- The larger the prosthesis, the more likely it is to interfere with nipple and skin sensation as a larger pocket has to be dissected and the nerves will be more stretched.

So, there is a battle here between size and form. Your surgeon can only try and advise you, ultimately it is *your* choice.

MEASURING THE SIZE OF PROSTHESIS

One of the ways of doing this is for the patient to bring in a sports bra with a cup that they aspire to fill. The surgeon can then fill the cup with sizing prostheses and come up with a reasonable estimate as to what prosthesis should be used. Of course this is inaccurate in as much as it all depends on how hard the prosthesis is stuffed into the cup. A prosthesis placed under the muscle tends to produce a slightly smaller increase in size.

3D PHOTOGRAPHY AND COMPUTER MORPHING

It is now possible for you to have a photograph taken of your breast by computer simulation with a new breast created. This mimics the likely outcome following surgery and allows for volume to be estimated in the breast area. You will have the chance to see your current shape versus the one you aspire to be from various angles that you may not have seen before.

FURTHER DETAILS YOU MAY WISH TO DISCUSS WITH YOUR SURGEON

Incisions:

ARMPIT (AXILLARY)
- Only for the first operation
- Prosthesis must be sub-muscular
- Usually done with endoscopic assistance
- This indirect approach can result in an increased need for adjustments.

AROUND THE AREOLA (PERIAREOLAR)
- Limited approach
- Sometimes scars very good
- Sometimes scars highly visible
- May alter nipple sensation.

SUBMAMMARY
- Best if any asymmetry present
- Anatomical implants can only be inserted through this incision
- At present the preferred incision because access to

the pocket is direct, with less postoperative pain. There is also less risk of capsular contracture
- Best for biplanar procedures
- Part of the ABBA Technique (*see also* page 149).

There are several positions for pockets (see below).

IN FRONT OF THE PECTORAL MUSCLE (SUBGLANDULAR)
- Less painful
- Prosthesis more easily seen, especially if thin
- Increased rates of capsular contraction
- Increased loss in nipple sensation
- Breast more likely to drop with the weight
- Induces more loss of natural breast tissue.

UNDER THE PECTORAL MUSCLE (SUBMUSCULAR)
- Preferred pocket of many surgeons
- More padding to disguise the prosthesis
- Less likely to interfere with nipple sensation
- Less capsule formation and better disguise if it occurs
- Less interference with mammograms
- May get unnatural movement
- Part of the ABBA Technique (*see also* page 149).

BIPLANAR OR DUAL PLANE
- A new operation to correct moderate droopiness
- The top half of the implant is under the muscle and the lower half is in front

- Allows correction of mild to moderate droop without the scars of a mastopexy procedure (*see also* Chapter 12).

SUMMARY

At the end of the consultation you should know about:
- The surgeon and his experience
- How the operation is performed
- Where the operation will be performed
- What type of anaesthetic is to be used
- Likely recovery and aftercare
- The risks and complications
- Your suitability and limitations (trade-offs and compromises)
- The aftercare
- Who pays for any complications
- Guarantees given with the prosthesis
- The cost.

If you are at all unsure, make sure you are offered a free second consultation with the surgeon.

THE BOTTOM LINE

All of the above will enable you to go away, digest the information and reflect before making the final decision, which is yours alone.

6

ANAESTHESIA

INTRODUCTION

Many women coming for breast augmentation will have concerns regarding the anaesthetic that they will receive, possibly because it is their first time or they may have had a bad experience in the past. Your anaesthetist is a doctor who will have undertaken five to eight years' further training after qualifying. He/she will visit you before the operation and it is a good idea to have any issues in your mind or written down to avoid forgetting anything before your preoperative visit. Your anaesthetist will spend time discussing with you the options available before you decide together on the best way to manage the anaesthetic and control the pain after surgery.

Modern anaesthesia is generally very safe; however, to

ensure that the best possible care is provided, it is important that you complete and return a health questionnaire before you arrive at the hospital (see Pre-Assessment, below).

The anaesthetic is an integral part of the operation. Your anaesthetist will see you for an assessment before the operation and remains with you throughout the operative procedure. He/she will make sure that you are comfortable and not in pain after the operation.

PRE-ASSESSMENT

Before deciding with your surgeon that you are to go ahead with breast augmentation, you will be asked to fill in a detailed health questionnaire. If you are taking medication or have any pre-existing lung, heart or kidney disease, you may be asked to have some routine blood tests, an ECG or chest X-ray. These are more likely to be called for if you are over sixty years old.

The purpose of the pre-assessment is to ensure all the information that your anaesthetist needs is ready on the day of surgery so delays and cancellations are avoided. If any abnormalities show up, then the pros and cons of proceeding may need to be explored again. It is important to be open about any special problems you may have; in particular, high blood pressure, heart disease, breathing difficulties, diabetes and bleeding disorders. We also need to identify any medication that you may be taking. Most of the time we ask that you stay on the drugs until the day of your operation, but we must be aware of this in advance.

Special instructions are given if you have diabetes, are on anti-hypertensive therapy, antidepressants or have been treated with corticosteroids in the past.

We ask you not to take aspirin or aspirin-containing drugs prior to surgery (at least fourteen days before) as this can affect the ability of your blood to clot and you are more vulnerable to bleeding and haematoma formation.

PREPARATION FOR ANAESTHESIA

If you smoke, then this is a great opportunity to stop prior to surgery – it will lessen the chance of a chest infection and coughing in recovery. There is no need to give up alcohol entirely, but it is sensible to limit your alcohol intake in the lead-up to surgery. If you have not seen a dentist for a while, it is advisable to have any work done beforehand.

Have a good stock of painkillers that you know work and are tolerated by you. You will be given painkillers by the hospital, should you need them but your own will be cheaper.

Women on the contraceptive pill are safe to continue taking the drug, provided they are only having breast augmentation and will be staying in hospital for one day. If you are due to stay in hospital for a longer period, you are advised to stop taking the oral contraceptive pill (OCP) as oestrogenic hormones make the blood stickier and increase the risk of blood clots forming. Use alternative precautions and return to the pill at a later cycle.

If there is any suspicion that you may be pregnant, please take a pregnancy test and advise the medical staff straight away.

PREOPERATIVE VISIT

Shortly before surgery your anaesthetist will visit you in your room; they will have read your pre-assessment forms and if needed, checked your laboratory tests. Hopefully discussions will already have taken place between yourself, the surgeon and the anaesthetist with regard to how your anaesthetic will be managed. If not, this is the time to express any concerns you may have. Your anaesthetist will go over your medical and surgical history then examine you, if necessary, to make an assessment of your airway.

PREMEDICATION

The practice of premedicating patients has largely ceased. In the past this was used to reduce the unpleasant actions of the drugs and gases required for anaesthesia. Modern anaesthetics are fast, efficient, comfortable and non-irritant. It is normal to feel anxious and nervous prior to an operation. If you are extremely anxious then a sedative such as Temazepam may help. However, these can also cause drowsiness and may slow down your recovery after the operation.

PREOPERATIVE 'NIL BY MOUTH'
Were you to be sick during an anaesthetic this could be extremely dangerous to your health as the acid stomach contents can pass into the lungs so there are special rules that we insist patients adhere to. You must starve yourself for at least six hours before surgery in order to empty your stomach. This means *no food*. If you need to swallow some pills, water is permitted. Modern-day surgery guidelines allow/encourage clear fluids (i.e. water or a carbohydrate sports drink up to two hours pre-op).

- Operations in the morning: Ideally, you should starve from midnight.
- Operations in the afternoon: You may have a light breakfast at 6am, but nothing afterwards.
- Uncertain of your exact time? We suggest you starve yourself from midnight.
- Even if you are having a local anaesthetic you may need to starve in case it becomes necessary to put you to sleep or to use sedation.
- If your operation has to be performed for an emergency (for example, haematoma evacuation) and you have not starved, do not worry: we have special ways of dealing with this and can explain at the time, should this very rare need arise.

- A good rule of thumb is not to have any food or milky drinks for six hours prior to a general anaesthetic.

DIFFERENT TYPES OF ANAESTHESIA
Local Anaesthesia

Your surgeon injects a local anaesthetic (often lignocaine) into the tissues that are to be operated on. You will stay conscious throughout the procedure, just as you would when visiting the dentist and having part of the jaw numbed, though for a breast augmentation far more local anaesthetic will be required. Your surgeon will need to inject a large volume of local anaesthetic under the skin and deeper tissues at many points so the breast is sufficiently numb to allow surgery to begin. He/she may also block several nerves running between your ribs (intercostal nerves) to provide the best effect. This process is extremely uncomfortable and it is often the case that during surgery supplementary local anaesthetic will need to be injected.

For these reasons, performing breast augmentation purely with local anaesthetic is rarely attempted as it is too uncomfortable for most women to tolerate. However, local anaesthesia is likely to form an important part of the overall anaesthetic management plan as it helps to control postoperative pain. Local anaesthesia can be combined with sedation or general anaesthesia and its skilled application means you will need less of the sedating agents, resulting in a faster recovery after surgery.

Regional Anaesthesia

With regional anaesthesia large areas of the body are numbed by the application of local anaesthetic agents to large nerves or to the spinal cord. The most common example would be a woman who receives an epidural to ease the pain of childbirth or to undergo a caesarean section. She will remain conscious, but pain-free throughout the procedure.

Theoretically, breast augmentation could be performed under epidural but with the injection being placed much further up the spinal column. In practice, though, the risks to breathing and circulation would be too great, so regional anaesthesia is unlikely to be part of your overall management.

Intravenous Sedation

Sedation alone is insufficient for breast augmentation; it needs to be combined with local anaesthesia. If you should decide to have intravenous sedation you will receive one, two or possibly three sedating agents into a cannula (small needle) that is placed into your arm by the anaesthetist. The agents may be given continuously (i.e. by infusion) or intermittently (by bolus – in one hit rather than via a gradual drip). When sedated, you become relaxed and sleepy, entering a twilight state, where you are likely to fall asleep and remember little of surgery. However, it should be possible to rouse you at any time by shouting your name. You might awaken briefly as an uncomfortable part of the surgery is performed – for instance, the first injection of local anaesthetic under the skin or as the prosthesis is inserted.

General Anaesthesia

Receiving a general anaesthetic means that you will be unconscious for the operation and will feel nothing; you will not be woken by any means during the procedure. A general anaesthetic has two components: induction (sending you into unconsciousness) and maintenance (keeping you unconscious until the end of the operation).

Intravenous agents normally provide induction (most commonly Propofol, which is recognisable by its milky appearance), though it is possible to induce anaesthesia by breathing an anaesthetic vapour instead. Known as 'gaseous induction', it is normally intended for small children but an option to be discussed with your anaesthetist if you have serious needle phobia as it can be performed without having a cannula in place.

Maintenance will ordinarily be provided by anaesthetic gases such as nitrous oxide (laughing gas) and Sevoflurane. Towards the end of the operation the anaesthetist will stop administering the gases and you will breathe air and oxygen to enable you to wake up.

In recent years it has been increasingly common to maintain anaesthesia with intravenous agents.

Total Intravenous Anaesthesia (TIVA)

TIVA is general anaesthesia provided by continuous infusion(s) of anaesthetic agent(s). Propofol is the standard agent used but often the anaesthetist will give a second infusion of an opiate – a drug with a morphine-like action to help with pain. Opiates such as Alfentanil or Remifentanil, however, have a much shorter duration of action than morphine, so when the anaesthetist stops their infusion you will wake up with a little hangover feeling.

In practice there is no sharp cut-off between intravenous sedation and TIVA; your anaesthetist is using the same agents, but at different rates. Propofol infused at a slow rate will provide twilight sleep; given much faster, it produces general anaesthesia in which your anaesthetist will need to take control of your breathing.

In the best hands using TIVA can result in lower rates of nausea and vomiting and a faster recovery from your anaesthetic, so you may spend less time in recovery and are fit to go home sooner than if you had received anaesthetic gases.

TRANSFER TO THEATRE

After all the necessary preparations have been completed on the ward you will be walked to the operating theatre anaesthetic room. It is perfectly acceptable for a close relative or friend to come along with you. You will be asked to lie down on a trolley and a number of simple devices will be attached to your body to enable us to monitor your blood pressure, check on your heart tracing and also confirm the amount of oxygen being delivered to your tissues. This is completely normal and enables us to provide the highest-quality care for you at all times.

After this has been performed a small needle (cannula) will be inserted into a vein, either on the back of your hand or in the forearm. If you are particularly frightened of needles or hate injections, we can numb the skin with a special anaesthetic cream but it must be applied one hour before the operation so you must let the anaesthetist know.

Alternatively, you may ask to be put to sleep with anaesthetic gas. You will be requested to take several deep breaths of oxygen and gas. Before you know it, you will be asleep.

When you are asleep, it is quite common to set up an intravenous infusion of fluid (a drip) to replace fluid lost during the operation and to make up for the fluid you did not drink while being starved. In the very unlikely event that we have to give you a blood transfusion, we can use the same drip.

RECOVERY WARD AFTER SURGERY

When the operation is complete you will be transferred from the operating table onto your bed and moved into recovery. The nursing staff will closely monitor you for between thirty and sixty minutes, during which time you will be given some oxygen to breathe and be provided with additional painkillers and anti-sickness medicine, as required. Thereafter you will return to the ward to complete your stay.

RISKS OF ANAESTHESIA

Anaesthesia today is safe due to advances in drugs, equipment and the training of the anaesthetists. However, like almost anything in modern life there are risks attached to having an anaesthetic. Your anaesthetist will stay with you throughout the whole procedure, ready to quickly and effectively intervene should the need arise. Of course if you are having a general anaesthetic you won't be aware of this. With pre-existing medical conditions the risks are increased and it is sensible to discuss them with your surgeon and anaesthetist well before the date of the operation.

The chances of you dying are quoted as 1:100,000. However, since most women undergoing breast augmentation are fit and well (being treated as a day case), the risk is less and probably nearer to one in half a million.

Postoperative Nausea and Vomiting (PONV)

About one in three patients having a general anaesthetic will experience nausea (an intense feeling of queasiness) or vomiting. Women are more prone to this than men, but breast augmentation surgery in itself is relatively low risk compared to, say, gynaecological or ear surgery.

It is likely that you will routinely be given one anti-emetic (a drug to counteract PONV), often Ondansetron. However, if you are high risk because of previous PONV after surgery or have bad travel sickness, you may be given a second or third anti-emetic such as Dexamethasone (a steroid) or Cyclizine (an anti-histamine).

It is worth making your anaesthetist aware of any previous PONV as they may alter their anaesthetic technique to minimise the chances of reoccurrence.

Damage to your teeth or mouth

There is a 1:4,500 chance of your teeth being damaged during the course of an anaesthetic. The risk increases if you have abnormalities such as loose teeth, protruding incisors, reduced mouth opening or neck movement.

It is important that you tell your anaesthetist about any abnormalities so care can be taken to avoid damage; you must also mention any expensive dental bridgework or veneers that could be damaged. You may have a plastic tube inserted into your mouth to ensure breathing remains unobstructed while you are asleep.

This process may knock and damage a vulnerable tooth (very rare).

For the same reason, there is a 1:20 chance of a small scratch or bruise to your lips or tongue. These heal quickly and may be helped by applying some Vaseline.

Sore throat

This is the most common side effect of a general anaesthetic and there is a 40 per cent chance of having a sore throat, but most breast augmentations can be managed with a less traumatic tube called a 'laryngeal mask' (LM). Insertion of a LM reduces the risk of a sore throat to 20 per cent. In either case symptoms normally resolve within two days.

Shivering

Under anaesthetic your core body temperature will drop, resulting in shivering as you awaken. This can be disturbing, but it is harmless. To avoid shivering, theatre staff will probably wrap you in a blanket warmed by hot air. It also helps to come to theatre warm and your anaesthetist will welcome this as your veins stand out.

If these measures fail and you are still shivering, there are drugs such as low doses of Pethidine, which can alleviate this. As long as you are receiving oxygen, shivering is not dangerous and will pass within thirty minutes.

Awareness

One of the most common fears is that of being awake or aware during surgery and feeling pain, but not being able to do anything about it. Some high-profile cases in the media caused alarm in many.

The most recent study in the UK at the time of writing showed an overall risk of 1:14,000 of being aware during surgery. Breast augmentation has an even lower risk since it is unlikely that you will be required to be paralysed for the operation and it is the paralysing agents that the anaesthetist gives for some types of surgery that result in the patient being unable to move to show their distress. Occasionally, if the implant is placed under the pectoralis muscle, then the surgeon will ask the anaesthetist to paralyse the patient so that the muscle relaxes to aid placement of the implant.

Your anaesthetist will monitor the level of the gases that you are receiving and your pulse, breathing rate and blood pressure to alert him/her to any early signs of awareness. If you are having TIVA they may also analyse your brain waves with a BIS monitor to ensure you are asleep, although this is not in universal use.

Allergic reactions

If you have previously had allergic reactions, ranging from skin rashes to life-threatening anaphylaxis, then the nurse admitting you will place a warning bracelet on your wrist and you will be asked on several occasions to confirm your allergy history.

There is a very low risk of today's anaesthetic agents causing a serious allergic reaction but some patients will react to intravenous antibiotics (given to prevent the implant from getting infected), latex in gloves or paralysing drugs, should they be needed.

Remember, your anaesthetist is well trained in treating allergic reactions and you are in a safe environment with all the necessary drugs to counteract the reaction, should it occur in the operating room.

Thrombosis and Embolism

While undergoing surgery, other risks include thrombosis. 'Deep Vein Thrombosis' (DVT) occurs as a result of abnormal clotting in a large vein, normally in the leg. The leg may become hot, swollen and painful. Should the clot dislodge, it would travel in the circulation to the lungs called 'pulmonary embolism' (PE) and is potentially life threatening.

We have learnt that it is neither the anaesthetic nor the operation per se that is the cause, but long periods of immobility (exactly the same as those rare cases of passengers on long-haul flights who do not move at all out of their seats). As a result we mobilise our patients early. Given that breast augmentation generally takes one to one-and-a-half hours, it is rarely a problem but there is a slightly increased risk if you smoke and/or take a contraceptive pill high in oestrogens or HRT.

To lower the risk of DVT/PE you are given tight socks to wear for theatre and your calves will be gently compressed to maintain circulation. If your surgeon or anaesthetist thinks you are at a higher risk of DVT/PE, you may be given an anticoagulant injection for a few days after leaving hospital.

Chest infection
Very occasionally, a chest infection may occur. This is far more common in smokers and those with lung disease.

POSTOPERATIVE PAIN
We cannot promise there will be no pain. You will certainly experience some discomfort after undergoing breast augmentation. A feeling of chest constriction or tightness is the most common complaint but this soon passes.

Your likelihood of acute pain depends on the following:
• How much local anaesthetic your surgeon uses
• How much analgesia the anaesthetist gives you while you are asleep and in recovery
• Your personal pain threshold
• How large your implants are and whether your breasts have already been stretched by pregnancy and breastfeeding.

Most anaesthetists will give sufficient analgesia so that when you are moved from the operating theatre to recovery, you simply have to wake up before going back to your room. Sometimes the recovery nurse will give you additional analgesia (most often morphine) to make you comfortable. The nurse administers small frequent doses until you say the pain is controlled.

You will probably be given a Paracetamol and Codeine combination such as Tylex or Co-dydramol to take home. Some patients may be given Ibuprofen (Nurofen) or Diclofenac (Voltarol). Though effective, there is greater risk of postoperative bleeding so some avoid use. Hence it is very useful to already know what works for you and can be tolerated.

THE BOTTOM LINE
Most breast augmentations are performed under general anaesthesia or TIVA as a day case.

Finally, our frequently asked questions (FAQs) and answers concerning anaesthesia may be found at the back of this book under Further Information (*see* page 221).

7

RISKS AND COMPLICATIONS

The only surgeon who does not have any complications is the one who does not operate. Risks and complications are the unforeseen and unplanned adverse effects of any surgical procedure that neither the patient nor the surgeon wishes. It is important to understand that all surgeons have them, but the best tend to have fewer.

Be aware that you will have:
- Swelling
- Bruising
- A feeling of tightness across the chest
- A different sensation in the breast and nipple-areola complex (NAC)
- A more obvious/erect nipple.

These are not complications, but an inevitable part of any breast augmentation. You may also experience a sensation of air and/or water crackling or slopping around for the first few days or weeks.

Forewarned about the possibility of a complication, you can at least accept it. If not, patients tend to view it as if something has gone wrong and any explanation is an excuse. This represents additional time and anxiety for both patient and surgeon. Difficulties occur with even the best precautions and surgical technique. It is more a test of your surgeon how he/she deals with any complication compared to a simple and uncomplicated case, allowing you to become even more trusting of them.

A complication does not always spell disaster and may simply delay your initial healing. Often the long-term result may be indistinguishable from a patient who did not experience any complications.

Complications may be attributable to:
• Anaesthesia
• Surgery
• Implant.

Anaesthesia
Modern methods of anaesthesia are immensely safe and the risks and complications have already been detailed in the previously chapter.

RISKS AND COMPLICATIONS

Surgery

As part of their duty of care, surgeons should always mention to prospective patients complications that are either common or 'significant'. The issue is deciding at what level to draw the line: should we have multiple pages of every conceivable complication, as in the US, and risk missing the rare one that, because it happens to you and you alone, is highly significant? A common level chosen is 1 per cent (1:100) or above but so many studies give different figures and individual surgeons might be different anyway, so it is impossible to be precise. An approximate guide has 'infrequent', 'rare' and 'very rare'.

Infrequent

SCARRING

If a surgeon cuts the skin with a scalpel, a scar will result, bleeding occurs and infection is possible. The overwhelming majority of scars will heal normally and give no problem whatsoever. Coloured skin has a higher risk of developing hypertrophic or keloid scarring. These are forms of excess scar formation; the former are confined to the incision, and settle down with time or simple treatment, such as pressure or steroid injection. The latter last a long time, extend beyond the boundaries of the original incision and are hard to treat. It is fortunate that their presence in the fold beneath the breast is rare.

Unless you have previously undergone surgery and paid close attention to how your scar changed over time, you will probably be unaware of the biological process of scar maturation. Initially, scars are very faint and difficult to see, but rapidly worsen as they become red and raised. This is entirely normal and simply indicates that the body is healing normally. It takes up to one year for the final result of how a scar looks and feels.

HAEMATOMA

A collection of blood within the pocket is known as a 'haematoma'. With modern techniques, more likely it may be caused during insertion of the rough-surfaced implants than poor surgical technique. It shows itself as a progressive swelling of the breast, usually one side, and increasing tightness and pain. If left, it gives a much higher rate of formation of a capsular contracture (see below). Bleeding usually occurs within the first few hours of surgery and is the main reason for patients either staying in hospital overnight or taking a room in a local hotel if they live some distance away. It is remedied by the simple procedure of a brief anaesthetic, clot removal and re-suturing of the wound.

ASYMMETRY

This is an issue that can cause postoperative distress, but can be avoided if comprehensive examination and assessment has been performed prior to surgery. When questioned, most women are aware of their own two breasts being different in some way, but others have never noticed. This may be a situation that is improved with an augmentation – in some cases different sizes are used on each side – but do remember that nature is rarely perfectly symmetrical and it is normal to have some degree of difference between the two breasts. A new technology is becoming available to assist with implant selection: 3D photography is both highly accurate and a great help in visualising the situation because a 3D image is taken of your own chest. Different computer-generated implant options can then be shown and surgeons are finding it very helpful in matching breasts with more than a slight difference. It is also common for women to have chest wall asymmetries also and this will certainly impact on the final look of the augmented breast (*see* Fig.6). Be aware that small differences may be magnified by breast enhancement surgery.

Depression

While we are not suggesting that breast augmentation causes women to become psychologically unhinged, there is a recognition that some pass through a bit of a 'dip' in the weeks after surgery. There is no evidence that it is some organic, psychiatric diagnosis, but something that invariably passes quickly. It may be a consequence of the general anaesthetic or, perhaps more likely, a feeling of anti-climax at the longed-for BA actually being complete. Of course the breasts are swollen and feel very strange at first, so it is probably no great surprise. Rest assured, it soon passes.

CAPSULAR CONTRACTURE

Just as any incision made in human skin results in a scar, a similar process occurs in the dissected pocket made for the implant, where the body forms a protective layer of scar tissue that covers the prosthesis. This is a standard biological reaction that occurs when any foreign matter is inserted into the human body, be it artificial joints, cardiac valves, contraceptive implants or breast implants. In fact, this fibrous bag, or 'capsule' provides an extra layer of protection in the event of implant shell failure.

A problem occurs if the capsule is unusually active and contracts enough to produce a feeling of hardness, distortion and, occasionally, pain. This is known as 'adverse capsular contracture' (ACC), 'hardening' or 'rejection' (an inaccurate term, but one which appears on the internet). Twenty years ago, rates were of the order of 50 per cent: yes, one in two. Today, though not yet zero, it is well below 10 per cent and some techniques, including ABBA (American anti-Biotic Breast Augmentation), have rates at the 2 per cent level. To reiterate: not yet zero, but much improved.

A capsule that distorts the final result can either be left and the result accepted or surgery may be attempted to rectify the situation. It is important to appreciate that having had a contracted capsule makes one more likely to experience a recurrence and there are a tiny number of women who seem to form capsules and may not be suited to breast implants in the long term. They may be advised to use polyurethane covered implants instead.

Rare
SEROMA
Just as blood may collect in the pocket around the prosthesis so may fluid (seroma) that produces swelling and, extremely rarely, may require drainage. It declares itself through swelling and/or pain, usually some time after surgery.

MALPOSITION/MALROTATION
Modern, textured (rough-coated) implants are believed to partially 'stick' to the body's tissues, which makes the likelihood of them changing position far less frequent than in days gone by, when smooth-shelled implants were en vogue. Of course, if a round one rotates, it will not be noticed but the same is not true for anatomically shaped versions that will produce breast distortion, if displaced. Good surgical technique is important in the prevention of malposition and malrotation.

FURTHER ('MAINTENANCE') SURGERY
Difficult to precisely define, although we have moved

away from advising planned replacement of breast prostheses on a ten-year basis. If you live long enough, it is likely that some future surgery will be required. While previously this was often precipitated by a ruptured implant, modern prostheses are markedly improved and it may have become more likely that surgery (known as 'maintenance') will be due to the breast changing around the implant, e.g. continued ageing produces ptosis (droop). The rupture rate of the latest fifth generation implants in recent studies sits around 1–6 per cent over the first ten years. You actually play an important role in determining this through your choice of implant size: if they are much larger than your natural tissue envelope, you'll be heading for a mastopexy (uplift) sooner rather than later.

SENSATION
Sensitivity and nipple erectability are highly variable in the general population; therefore, the consequences of augmentation are equally varied. We can almost guarantee that there will be some change, usually a diminished sensation, in the early postoperative period that should return to normal over the following weeks and months. Others have an irritating increase in their sensation. The increased nipple erectability can be explained by the fact that a breast implant produces a firm and full breast upon which the NAC sits, and now sits more proud.

We know that placing the implant on top of the muscle risks more permanent changes to the nerves as they lie in the layer between breast and muscle. Also, we know most of the changes are due to nerve stretch so it follows that the bigger the implant, the more/longer the change in nerve function.

Nipple areola sensation, be it more or less often returns to normal with time. Commonly, patients have less feeling between the nipple areola and the incision.

Very rare

INFECTION

It is fortunate that infection is extremely rare. If it occurs it will not usually allow the implant to remain within the breast: either it will extrude (be pushed out) or have to be surgically removed. This is the same for any infected foreign body (e.g. hip or knee replacement), but doubly so as re-implantation is not usually attempted for three to six months. It usually affects only one side, thus causing a problem with clothes and the like. Although some have attempted salvage through hospitalisation, intravenous antibiotics and a fresh implant, this is rare; the standard regimen is implant removal, followed by healing and replacement when the infection and induration (the hard tissue that has not yet finished healing and may have active infection still on board) have completely cleared. A new implant must not be fitted until all signs of infection have passed. This may take up to six months.

PNEUMOTHORAX

Even less frequent is pneumothorax (a condition whereby air leaks out of the lung and into the chest cavity, causing the lung to collapse). While it may be a consequence of the surgery, it should not be so as the operation takes place on the outside of the ribcage and not inside but some patients, including asthmatics and thin people, are at risk of spontaneous lung collapse. It may also be related to air pressure as part of the anaesthetic ventilation. Whatever the cause, it is important to recognise and treat the condition, although if small, it may be left to resolve on its own. If larger, a chest drain may have to be inserted between the ribs, which will prolong hospitalisation and leave a small additional scar in the armpit.

There are other risks/complications less easily quantifiable, including the following.

BREASTFEEDING

There are no comparative studies of this subject. Firstly, research has shown silicone breast augmentation to be entirely safe for breastfeeding newborns. Secondly, there is much hoo-ha about implants stopping breast-milk production, but the logic is that women with implants are, in the main, small-breasted so less likely to be able to produce milk anyway. Placing the prosthesis beneath the muscle, via an IMF incision, has no physical basis for impairing the function of the breast unless of such a large size that it causes pressure effects on the glands.

PROMINENT VEINS

Being an active organ, the breast has a good blood supply, with arteries transporting fresh blood in and veins taking the used blood out. It is simply a matter of hydrostatics and pressure, whereby a large foreign body in the breast will squeeze the internal veins. Being highly adaptable, the body will see to it that the surface veins enlarge to allow for greater blood flow and you may notice more prominent veins on the outside. These mostly subside when the breast has become accustomed to the implant, but occasionally the external veins remain prominent: this is more likely with oversized prostheses. Although recorded in the literature and books, thrombosis of one or more superficial veins – a condition known as 'Mondor's disease' – is extremely rare. While uncomfortable, it is self-limiting and usually responds to simple anti-inflammatory drugs. Alternatively, the subcutaneous cords often running across the inframammary fold (IMF) can be snapped with firm finger pressure.

STRETCH MARKS

These occur whenever the skin is called upon to increase

either too quickly or too much. Most will have seen (or themselves be) a mother with some stretch marks (striae) as a reminder of pregnancy. Their presence depends on genetics, skin quality (especially elasticity) and size, or number, of pregnancies. The same is true of the breast: too much implant for the natural envelope elasticity will risk permanent stretch marks. By the same token, the nipple-areola complex (NAC) may appear to increase in size. This is partly due to the taking up of tissue elasticity, when the implant is inserted and some stretch. The latter will be proportionate to the implant and so the larger the size, the more the stretch.

CHRONIC PAIN

This indicates a pain either always present, or one that comes and goes many years after the surgery. While the occasional twinge is not unexpected, given the relative amount of foreign body moving about in the native breast, it is rare to have constant pain. If so, it is often associated with a change in shape and a capsular contracture. With older generation implants, leakage of the filler gel ('gel bleed') was often the cause, as was frank rupture. A very small proportion of patients are unfortunate enough to experience an ill-understood condition known as 'Chronic Regional Pain Syndrome' (CRPS). We are not entirely sure of the mechanism of CRPS, but it seems to involve some form of aberrant nerve regeneration and may occur after surgery in any area of the body; unfortunately some have it without having had surgery, just some blunt trauma. Fortunately, it is very rare after breast augmentation.

If you have managed to read through to this point, it may have struck you that many of the complications with BA relate to the chosen implant. They are to a large extent your choice, with advantages balanced against trade-offs, and should be discussed with your surgeon, who will advise accordingly.

Finally, your own self-image perception is an important and an ever-changing factor. Just as your body changes with time, so too will your mind!

THE BOTTOM LINE

- Don't go too large
- Use the ABBA Technique
- Sub-mammary incision
- Sub-muscular pocket
- Atraumatic pocket dissection
- Aseptic transfer of prosthesis
- Antibiotics for five days after surgery
- No drains (tubes that drain fluid from a wound)

8

THE BREAST PROSTHESIS

All breast implants are a silicone bag filled with either saline (essentially water with added salt) or silicone gel. The surface of the implant may be smooth or rough (textured), or covered in polyurethane.

Breast implants are surgical devices and although now closely regulated and tested, they are not perfect and do not last forever. They will create scar tissue (at the skin incision and around the pocket) and require maintenance at some stage. The length of time before maintenance is required is highly variable but all patients should expect to have further surgery in the future, either for an implant that has worn out or a breast that has changed (as they do with the passage of time and events such as pregnancy).

THE HISTORY OF SILICONE RELATED TO BREAST PROSTHESIS

In the late 1880s, British scientist Dr F.S. Kipping started experiments chemically combining carbon and silicon. The result was a sticky substance described at that time as resembling 'uninviting glue'! In the US, The Dow Corning Company used Dr Kipping's findings to invent silicone rubber in 1945. Silicone was a major discovery and when first invented was used to dampen the vibration of aircraft engines. After World War II, scientists concentrated on silicone's possible role in biology and medicine. Silicone was first used for medical purposes in 1953.

Medical-grade injectable silicone (known at the time as 'Dow Corning 200') was used in the 1950s and 1960s to enlarge female breasts, particularly in Asia. It soon became apparent, however, that liquid silicone was not a suitable substance as so much of it had to be used and it moved around. In those days, surgeons withdrew as much as 600ml (1 pint) from a 227-litre (50-gallon) drum and using a tool that resembled a large glue gun, shot the material under great pressure into the breast. In order to stop the silicone from moving about, an irritant such as paraffin or turpentine was added to provoke the body tissues into producing a protective reaction of inflammatory cells around the silicone, which helped keep it in place. In fact, what actually happened was that the silicone did not remain static where injected, but moved and usually exited as an infected mess through the skin. Having been injected under high pressure, it was not a discreet round ball, but a huge tumour often requiring the whole breast to be excised if it was to be completely removed!

The modern breast implant is based on an original implant introduced in 1962. It seems the idea happened on the spur of a moment when a plastic surgery resident at a leading USA hospital noticed one night in the blood-bank that the glass bottles used for storing blood had been replaced by silicone bags. After discussion with his chief, they decided to fill the silicone bag with liquid silicone producing a prototype breast prosthesis (it was not subjected to any medical testing).

A 28-year-old woman by the name of Timmie Jean Lindsey, attending the hospital to have a tattoo removed, was approached by the plastic surgeons and offered the chance to boost her bust. After six children, she had no hesitation in saying yes. Against all the odds, the implants remained in place for over forty years!

THE SILICONE SCARE

Silicone breast implants found themselves in a media spotlight in the 1990s when lawyers in the US claimed that silicone in the prosthesis caused:

• Breast cancer

- Abnormalities in babies born to mothers with silicone breast implants
- Autoimmune disease.

As a result of this, liquid silicone within the bag (but not the silicone bag itself) was withdrawn from use in the United States in 1994. Fortunately, the 'evidence' behind this has now been proven to be 'junk science' and the American FDA (Food and Drug Administration) cleared them for return to the market in December 2006. They were never withdrawn from use in the UK or many other European countries and so, unusually, the Americans find themselves behind Europe in this particular instance.

THE TRUE FACTS BEHIND SILICONE-FILLED BREAST PROSTHESIS

Silicone and breast cancer

In the twenty years since the moratorium on silicone breast implant use in the US, the various facts have become evident and agreed by the following:

- The UK government, who held an independent review in 1998 and re-confirmed their findings in 2004
- The FDA (Food and Drug Administration) in the US.

Fact: Women with silicone-filled breast implants have

no greater risk of breast cancer and some studies show a lower incidence of breast cancer than in women without implants.

Women who have had breast augmentation and develop breast cancer do not have a different prognosis to those without breast implants. It is believed that implants make palpation of tumours easier because they provide a firm surface underneath on which to feel any lumps.

Silicone breast implants do interfere with breast screening (mammography), so always advise your radiographer if you have implants. They can do different views to overcome the shadow (Eklund views). Squeezing of the breast should not rupture the prosthesis. Be aware that inserting the implants beneath the muscle allows more of the breast tissue to be visualised than under the gland.

Silicone and pregnancy

You can safely become pregnant and breastfeed! Even the most diehard Texan lawyers agree there is no link between women with breast augmentation and babies with a deformity, e.g. swallowing difficulties.

There is also no evidence that silicone implants are teratogenic (relating to, or producing, birth defects in babies). In fact, there is far more silicone in infant feeding formulae, teats and bottles than the breast milk of mothers with silicone breast implants.

Silicone and Autoimmune Connective Tissue Disease

Connective Tissue Disease (CTD) is a vague group of conditions covering a spectrum from ME to arthritis. There is no single X-ray or blood test to indicate whether or not you have CTD and so what the epidemiologists have done is to compare groups of women who have had silicone breast implants with control groups who have not had breast augmentation, all matched for age, race and previous medical problems.

There have now been thirty high-level published studies in peer reviewed journals. The bottom line is there is no difference between the two groups in developing diseases or symptoms and therefore in terms of health, silicone breast implants are considered safe.

Silicone gel implants have had to pass a detailed investigation held in 1998 by the Independent Review Group (IRG), commissioned by the British government at that time; it examined all the available evidence as to the safety of silicone breast implants. The investigation concluded there were no safety concerns; specifically, exposure to babies being breastfed by mothers with implants was no greater than those without implants. The panel met again in 2004 and found no new evidence that might allow them to alter their previous conclusions and recommendations.

THE MODERN PROSTHESIS
The prosthesis shell

Modern silicone implant shells, or elastomers have to undergo stringent testing by the European and American Regulatory Authorities for minimum standards of strength, durability and diffusion. Also, how much movement, pressure and creasing the prosthesis can withstand.

The elastomer is made with several layers, the best analogy being plywood. Typically, there are five layers, one of which has a special fluorinated treatment. This acts as a 'barrier' layer to specifically limit the leakage or 'bleed' of gel silicone through the wall of the prosthesis.

One of the problems with any foreign material inserted into the human body, including breast implants, is formation of a fibrous capsule of scar tissue around the implant. Because breast implants are not rigid (unlike metal joint replacements, for example), if the scar tightens then it can deform them. Surgeons know this as 'capsular contracture' but it is described more accurately on the internet as 'hardening' but also, inaccurately, as 'rejection'. Despite many decades of vigorous study, we still do not fully understand capsular contraction but the incidence has been markedly reduced from about 50 per cent to between 5 and 10 per cent today. A state-of-the-art review of what we currently know and understand about capsular contraction was published in 2011 and the latest 'ABBA Technique' suggests rates of 2 per cent. Although not yet zero, this is a massive reduction from 50 per cent.

Thirty years ago, implants coated in polyurethane foam were introduced, the idea being that the foam coating would break up the collagen fibres in the scar, leading to less capsular contracture than seen in the smooth surface implants used at that time. The reduction in capsular contracture rate was significant; however health concerns caused them to be banned: it was suggested that one of the breakdown products of polyurethane, 2-toluamine diamine (TDA), could cause cancer in mice.

Because it was realised that the polyurethane coating made such a difference, implant manufacturers decided to mimic the rough surface and so produced the 'textured' implant. There is controversy about the overall effect of texturing and the degree of texturing varies from manufacturer to manufacturer, indicating the final answer has not yet been provided. Textured surface implants have a lower risk of capsular contracture than smooth implants, but this is more pronounced with silicone gel than saline-filled implants. Anatomic implants are probably better with a textured surface as this will help maintain optimal positioning of the implant within its pocket.

Our experience shows that the precise type of texturing is important, too. Some implants seem to develop a second fibrous capsule ('pseudocapsule') around the prosthesis itself. It leads to an added problem because the pseudocapsule may contract and deform the overall result. This appears to be an intrinsic issue with the nature of the texturing itself rather than the real capsule.

Recently, the effect of polyurethane and its safety has been reassessed. We now have the benefit of experience of the 20,000 women in the United States and Europe who had polyurethane implants inserted twenty-five to thirty years ago and can conclude that there is no increased risk of breast cancer.

We believe that polyurethane-coated implants have a place, although we do not use them in primary breast augmentation but in some patients (either our own or other surgeons'), who have developed encapsulation and require removal of prosthesis and the capsule (capsulectomy). For severe or recurrent capsular contracture, we recommend reaugmentation with polyurethane-coated implants.

Saline-filled implants

You may have heard of saline-filled implants containing salt water rather than silicone gel and wonder why they are not used more often. Most experience of saline-filled implants is from the US: when silicone-filled implants were banned by the FDA (Food and Drug Administration) in 1994, American surgeons were left with no other option but to use saline implants for cosmetic purposes. They were still allowed to use silicone in reconstruction after breast cancer treatment, though. After many years of studies showing silicone gel implants to have no demonstrable health risks, the FDA (Food and Drug Administration) permitted their reintroduction in December 2006 for cosmetic purposes.

What are the experiences of saline-filled prostheses?
Saline-filled prostheses do not feel as natural as silicone gel prostheses. This depends on how much capsule formation there is around the prosthesis and how full they are filled.

Saline-filled prostheses have a higher rupture rate than gel-filled. There are two reasons for this:

- Manufacturers were keen that the prostheses should not be overfilled because they feared there would be an increased rupture rate and therefore the guarantee that they gave to their prostheses did not allow for overfilling. Unfortunately, if the prosthesis was not overfilled, then it had wrinkles.
- Saline is not as good a lubricant as silicone and therefore the movement of these folds led to cracking in the wall of the prosthesis and premature rupture. This rupture rate was not in any way dangerous as patients simply absorbed

the salt water. It proved hard on the patients'
bank account because they needed another
operation, though!

- Overall, saline-filled implants have slightly less
capsular contraction. However, recent studies
from the United States showed that up to 50
per cent of saline-filled prostheses have either
ruptured or require re-operation for other
reasons. Therefore the general
recommendation is to use silicone gel-filled
prostheses because they are safe, more
predictable and, depending on the amount of
capsule formation, more natural.

Silicone Gel Fillers

All silicone gels are 'cohesive', indicating a degree of
stickiness, but some are more cohesive than others so we
have two basic types: a liquid and semi-solid, cohesive
silicone gel. While the former can be poured, the latter
are able to retain their shape even with a ruptured shell,
but are a little firmer.

The latest fifth generation of highly viscous silicone
(known as 'form stable') has other advantages. In
addition to providing a shape to the implant they also
provide some resistance to capsular contracture and in
cases of rupture the silicone is less likely to migrate.
Removal after rupture is much easier with a cohesive gel
than a liquid gel implant.

Cohesive gel implants can be round or anatomical in shape. Round implants are designed on a round base and when properly filled, create a rounder appearance in the breast, with a fuller upper breast. If the implant is placed under the muscle, we can create a more natural-looking breast because the top half of the implant will be compressed more than the bottom half. However, if the implant is under-filled (much more likely to occur with saline filled prosthesis), then shell folding and wrinkling can occur, more likely leading to implant rupture.

This also means that the dissected pocket must be the right size for the implant. If an implant is squeezed into a pocket where the base is too small there will be an infolding of the implant wall right from the word go, which will lead to an increased risk of rupture. With anatomical implants, if the pocket is too large then the implant is free to move within the pocket and in the early stages may rotate or even flip over.

Anatomical shaped implants are shaped like a natural breast and some refer to anatomic implants as tear-drop implants.

HOW LONG WILL MY IMPLANT LAST?
How do we investigate the lifespan and rupture of an implant?
There are no set answers to these questions since the latest fifth-generation implants have only been available for a decade. The facts are these:

- Saline-filled implants have a greatly increased rupture rate and at five years, nearly 50 per cent of prostheses have had to be exchanged for one reason or another.
- The best study on silicone gel prostheses is by Per Hedén from Sweden, who showed that at seven years, 8 per cent of mixed generation prostheses had ruptured and most of these were asymptomatic. A more recent, but smaller study of fifth-generation implants showed that 99 per cent were intact after six years.

The longer your implants have been inserted, the more likely the chances of rupture. Therefore when we talk about a rupture rate or capsular contracture rate, we must clearly define how long the prosthesis has been in use. Different words are also used:

- Gel bleed: This is where the silicone shell of the prosthesis is intact but there is a slow diffusion of silicone gel across the wall. In almost every woman who has had a breast augmentation, a biopsy of the armpit lymph glands (to where the lymphatics of the breast mainly drain) would likely show some silicone on microscopic examination. There is no suggestion that this is in anyway significant, it is just the body's natural way of dealing with foreign substances. It is important to appreciate that gel bleed was a feature of the earlier generation implants but is now markedly reduced with the addition of the extra fluorinated layer in the shell of fourth- and fifth-generation implants.

- Gel leak: More significant from a practical viewpoint is rupture of the shell of the prosthesis. In many patients rupture, particularly with cohesive gel prostheses, is not thought to be significant – remember, your body has formed a protective fibrous capsule around the prosthesis and this will not wear out as it is being constantly replaced by normal scar repair mechanisms – and many women walk around completely unaware of their implants having ruptured. Others, however, may experience a burning sensation in the breast or a change in shape. A true change in volume is rare; an apparent change in size mostly occurs because women's breasts naturally become smaller with time.

If at some stage there is a significant change in your breast and its prosthesis, we can investigate this with:
- Clinical examination (cheap, but very inaccurate)
- Mammography (also inaccurate)

- An ultrasound (more accurate, but subject to operator-dependence)
- An MRI scan (the most expensive, but more accurate)
- Surgery (the only 100 per cent accurate method).

Should you be given a report of your ultrasound by the radiologist...

There are two forms of rupture with various ultrasound signs:

- **Intra-capsular** indicates that the prosthesis shell has broken, but silicone is contained by the body's scar capsule.
- **Extra-capsular** usually occurs as the result of heavy blunt trauma to the chest, producing rupture of both the prosthesis and the fibrous capsule around the prosthesis. Free silicone can now potentially migrate away from the breast and the armpit lymph glands may be enlarged from soaking it up. Most authorities recommend implant removal at this stage.

What should I do if my implant is ruptured?

Neither situation is considered dangerous. Many thousands of women walk around with ruptured prosthesis and they enjoy good health and have soft, normal shaped breasts. Others may have firm breasts but are happy with the situation, which they do not wish to change by a further operation.

To repeat, there is no evidence that a ruptured wall to your prosthesis in any way endangers your health and the so-called scare stories of silicone coming out in your hair and ears are a complete hoax.

WHAT FACTORS ARE INVOLVED IN CAUSING CAPSULAR CONTRACTURE?

- Haematoma
- Infection
- Silicone leak
- Time
- Fate (in other words, who knows?)

Many, many studies have looked into the reasons why capsular contracture occurs and we reviewed the medical evidence in 2011. Over the past two decades, the rate has been brought down from around 50 per cent to 5–10 per cent. We still do not fully understand why this occurs. The most unusual feature is the development of capsular contracture on only one side in most cases. So, we have the same patient, same implant (therefore patient-implant interface), same operation and same surgeon, so why it should occur on only one side is a mystery.

How can you lessen your chances of Capsular Contracture?
- Use a submammary incision allowing a subpectoral pocket with perfect haemostasis
- Use antibiotic washes and have five days of antibiotics afterwards (the ABBA technique)
- Do not use large prosthesis.

While the true figure for capsular contracture is probably in the order of 5–10 per cent, a technique developed by Dr Adams from the USA reports rates as low as 2 per cent over a six-year study period. This is the lowest figure we have found in our comprehensive review of the worldwide literature and we have adapted his technique, which we call 'ABBA':
- American
- anti-Biotic
- Breast
- Augmentation.

We have pioneered this technique in the UK and audit found our rates to be similar over the first two years.

Prosthesis companies
At the present time the major producers of breast implants are:
- NAGOR (British)
- Allergan (American) – formerly Inamed and McGhan

- MENTOR (American)
- SiliMED (originally Brazilian).

We have had a long association with Nagor and are happy to recommend their prosthesis. Last year, using the ABBA Technique, we had a 2 per cent encapsulation rate with the fifth-generation implants they have available.

IMPLANT GUARANTEES

Almost every company has a lifetime guarantee against rupture. Of course this is a slight con: the expensive part of having your implants replaced is not the implants themselves but the hospital and anaesthetist and possibly the surgeon's costs, depending on what arrangement you have. The implant guarantee is worth about 10 per cent of the total cost if the surgeon does not charge (and proportionately less if he/she does). What would be more appropriate with an implant guarantee is that the company pays for the whole operation of replacement and is not just providing you with free implants. It does, however, indicate that the implant manufacturers have sufficient confidence in their products to cover you for 100 per cent of the implant cost.

IMPLANT REMOVAL GUARANTEES

The fact that implants do not last a lifetime means

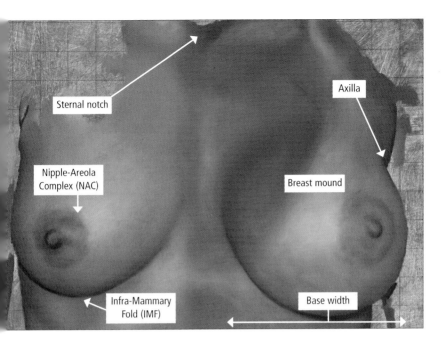

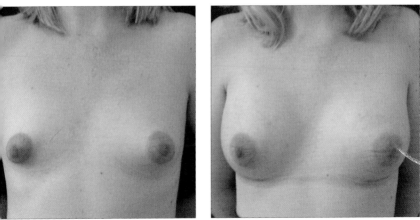

Figure 3 (*above*): main anatomical landmarks with a pre-operative breast on the left, augmented with an implant on the right.

*Images with kind permission of Jonathan Yeo (*You're Only Young Twice, *copyright 2011)*

Figure 4a (*below left*): a typical example of tubular breasts where a relatively normal-sized NAC is completely out of proportion with the underlying underdeveloped breast mound.

Figure 4b (*below right*): postoperative view at six months.

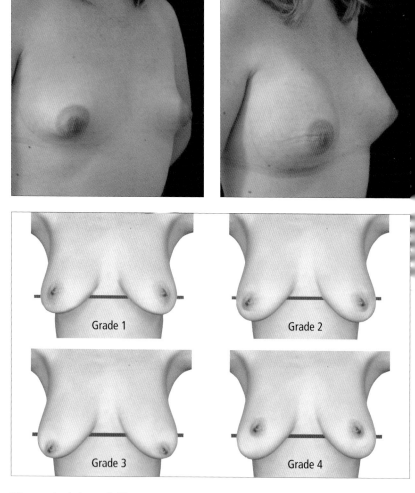

Figure 4c (*above left*): preoperative oblique angle showing the almost complete lack of projection of the breast mound, particularly in the lower parts.

Figure 4d (*above right*): appearance six months after a dual-plane augmentation. In this young patient the tissues are very tight and further stretch will occur over several months and assist with the curvature of the lower breast.

Figure 5 (*below*): degrees of ptosis (droop), which help determine the correct procedure.

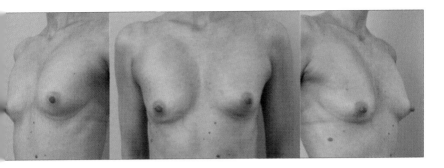

Figure 6: preoperative photographs of the case study showing differences in both the two breasts and each side of the chest.

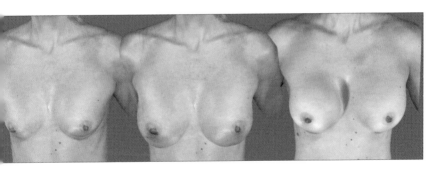

Figure 7: sequence of 3D representations with the pre-operative situation of the left. The centre has a 320cc implant on the right and 220cc on the left. Volumes have increased to 375cc and 290cc respectively on the right and this was the final combination selected for surgery.

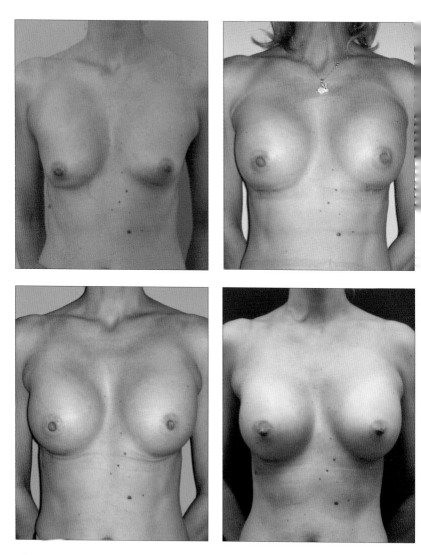

Figure 8a (*above left*): preoperative image.

Figure 8b (*above right*): photograph after one week where the slight redness is due to the dressings having just been removed.

Figure 8c (*below left*): after six weeks.

Figure 8d (*below right*): the patient remains delighted with her result after 12 months, but this series shows how much time and patience is required and it is especially difficult in the early period.

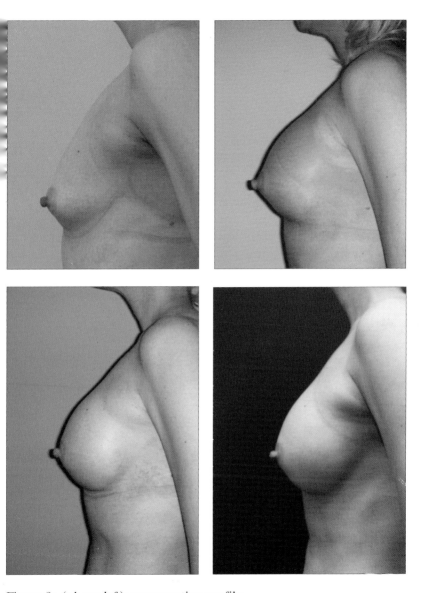

Figure 9a (*above left*): preoperative profile.

Figure 9b (*above right*): after first week.

Figure 9c (*below left*): after six weeks.

Figure 9d (*below right*): the profile view with settling of the tissues and final result after 12 months.

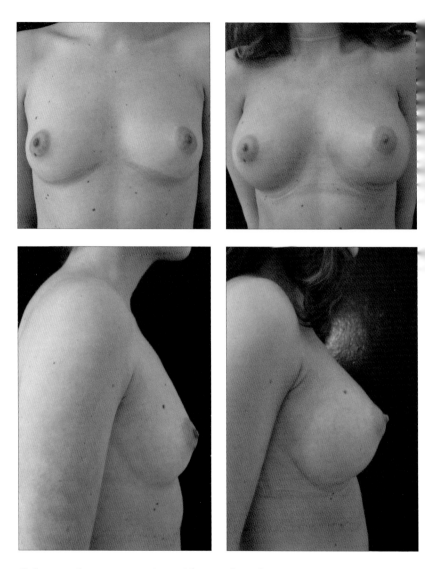

Submuscular augmentation with round implants.

Figure 10a (*above left*): preop of a young woman with an A cup.

Figure 10b (*above right*): six months after submuscular augmentation with a round implant and now a full C cup.

Figure 10c (*below left*): preop profile of above patient.

Figure 10d (*below right*): post-operative six month profile.

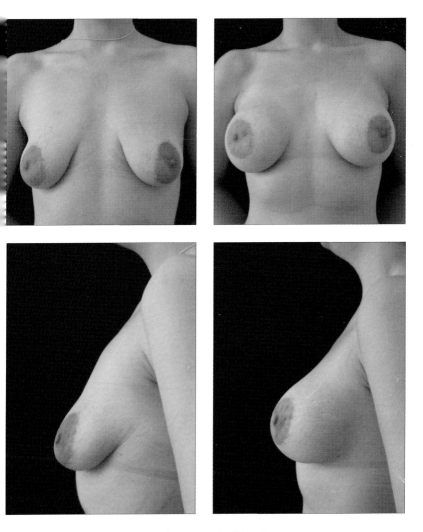

Dual-plane augmentation with anatomical implants.

Figure 11a (*above left*): a middle-aged woman who felt her breasts had drooped and lost volume after breastfeeding her two children. She wished to avoid the scars of an uplift (mastopexy).

Figure 11b (*above right*): following dual-plane augmentation with anatomical implants.

Figure 11c (*below left*): the same woman in profile view.

Figure 11d (*below right*): following anatomical dual-plane augmentation.

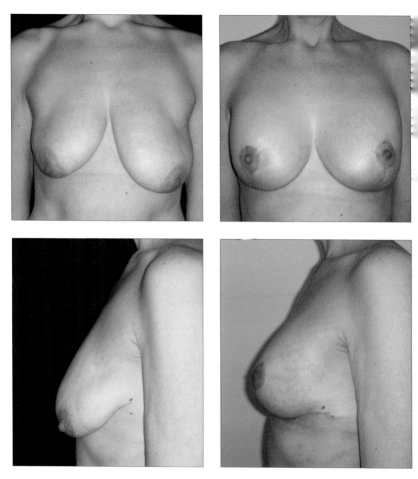

Augmentation-mastopexy.

Figure 12a (*above left*): a woman with not only droop and a loss of volume in the upper breast, but a significant asymmetry.

Figure 12b (*above right*): frontal view six months after augmentation-mastopexy with a round implant placed in a pocket beneath the muscle and 'anchor pattern' scarring.

Figure 12c (*below left*): lateral preop view showing the nipple at the lowest part of the breast (Grade 3 ptosis).

Figure 12d (*below right*): lateral photograph at six months. The nipple-areola complex has been lifted to a better position at the most projected part of the augmented breast.

further surgery ('maintenance') may need to take place in the future. When initially consulting the surgeon, you should ask about the lifespan of the implants you have chosen and also study the patient information literature accompanying your chosen implants. We recommend all patients having breast prosthesis fitted have a cohesive gel. It is a maxim of surgery that whatever is implanted should be easily and completely removable – and that is certainly true of cohesive silicone gel.

REGULATIONS

Breast prostheses are regulated in the UK by the 1993 European Medical Devices Directory and 2002 National UK Law; also in America by the FDA (the Food and Drug Administration), which performs the same regulatory function.

There are four classes of medical devices according to risk in the EC. In 2003, breast implants were reclassified to the highest (level 3) in order to bring all European implants in line with the UK.

The Conformité Européenne (CE) marketing is a manufacturer's declaration that the product complies with the health, safety and environmental requirements of the relevant product directive. It is a mark of quality assurance and allows free trade throughout Europe, though this is not required for export. The recent PIP debacle demonstrated that this system could not protect against the defective French implant, which was used by most of the cheaper cosmetic clinics. However, it did prove the old adage that 'you get what you pay for'.

THE BOTTOM LINE: PROSTHESIS

For primary first time augmentation, we believe that a cohesive gel with textured surface is the best available implant. This may be round or anatomical, depending on personal circumstances and preference.

For augmentation-mastopexy, i.e. where the breast needs to be lifted up in combination with an implant to add volume, we believe that a round textured cohesive gel implant is appropriate.

For patients presenting for secondary surgery with capsule formation we believe that a round polyurethane-coated implant is the best option for trying to prevent re-encapsulation.

WHAT ARE THE ALTERNATIVES TO THE USE OF SURGICAL BREAST PROSTHESES?
Exercise
In particular, bulking up the pectoralis major muscle. This will have a minor effect on the base upon which your breast rests and cannot have any effect on the breast itself. In fact, with the loss of weight that accompanies regular exercise, the breast may even shrink further.

Creams and drugs

There are hundreds of creams and homeopathic drugs which claim to increase the size of the breast. None have been adequately subjected to rigorous scientific testing. Any chemical that causes a degree of local inflammation will provoke some swelling of the breast, but this will be purely temporary and is hardly a safe and recommended course of action.

Free injection of liquid silicone

This has a very long and sad history. Medical grade silicone has been injected into, or under the breast, to increase its volume and was particularly common in Japan. The problem is that medical grade silicone is, on the whole, pretty inert and therefore it does not stay where it is injected. It has to be mixed with something that will cause inflammation, which in turn causes fibrous tissue, which will then fix the silicone. Paraffin and turpentine were top of this list and there were two consequences: firstly, a local reaction. Secondly, the inflammation/infection led to the body trying to expel the silicone, resulting in ulceration of the breast and some truly horrific deforming results. The silicone became extremely hard and painful and started to extrude, having been injected under force. Following this, the only method of treatment was removal of the breast itself (i.e. a mastectomy, as performed for cancer).

Suction

Recently, a system has been introduced from the United States called BRAVA that uses suction on the breast base and claims volume increases. While only small increases are seen, a breast volume increase has been proven by MRI scans. One problem is that it must be applied for twelve hours a day over a period of several months; another difficulty is making a good seal between the device and the suction ring so there are problems with both getting the BRAVA cup fitted and keeping it applied to the chest wall all night as it can cause ulceration and skin problems. The principal problem is that the expansion is not maintained. Once suction ceases, the breasts start to lose volume again.

Fat grafts

Recently the BRAVA system has been supplemented by free fat grafts and stem cells. Essentially, the breast is expanded with suction and then harvested fat is injected. Good, lasting results have been claimed and it may be that the blood supply is improved by suction. While in principle an attractive concept, there are still several issues:

- Most women who desire breast augmentation have little 'spare' fat that can be used.
- It takes several hours of theatre time and a team of staff to harvest, prepare and re-inject

the fat. In 2010, a 'two-in-one' procedure was widely trumpeted in the media by one of the companies but quickly sank into obscurity as a result of the significant extra cost.

- There is a limitation in the quantity of fat that can be safely transplanted at any one time of the order of a single cup size or so, thus multiple procedures are required.

- With transfer of fat comes growth factors and there remain concerns as to the long-term effect of these growth stimulators on a cancer-prone organ such as the breast. Studies are ongoing in women who already have cancer, but the bottom line is that we cannot be entirely certain it is safe.

- Any intervention in the breast leaves some form of scarring, which may take the form of microcalcifications. These small deposits of calcium show up on mammograms. A feature of benign and cancer disease, they may result in unnecessary biopsy, surgery and anxiety.

THE BOTTOM LINE

Fat injections are being used as part of breast reconstruction following cancer and while this procedure has been enthusiastically greeted by plastic surgeons, whether or not it is truly a major

---

breakthrough only time will tell. Unless they specifically do not wish to have a silicone prosthesis fat injection, this remains an expensive alternative for the average patient, with no long-term history of its safety or effectiveness at the time of writing.

9

PREPARATION FOR SURGERY

Here, we list some things you will need to consider and do in preparation for your breast augmentation. This list is compiled from various sources: firstly, what we as surgeons believe to be important and secondly, points made by previous patients (*see also* Chapter 14), whose helpful feedback has greatly assisted us in the preparation of this book.

GET TO KNOW YOUR BREASTS

Ensure that you are familiar with your breasts. If you are not already doing so – and it is important for all women to check their breasts regularly for abnormalities – you should perform breast self-examination each month just after your menstrual period or on the first day of each month after the menopause. This allows you to get used to the texture and feel of your breasts with any normal lumpiness; you will then have a good idea of what is part of you and your normal variation before surgery.

Equally important is the fact that you should note any asymmetry in your breasts and chest wall before surgery. No woman's breasts are perfectly identical and preoperative asymmetry is frequent – for instance, a nipple-areola complex (NAC) a little lower on one side than the other. It is important to understand that there is a great degree of variation in what is considered 'normal'. Commonly, and usually completely unnoticed, is that your shoulder may be carried higher on one side compared to the other, or that the inframammary fold (IMF) is at a different height. The width of your chest may also differ in size or contour – i.e. the ribs being more prominent on one side. All these factors should be considered before surgery with natural close inspection. After surgery, your chest may make you draw the wrong conclusion that it is the surgeon or the implants themselves that caused the asymmetry, not the fact that it was present before the operation. Breast augmentation is an operation on the breasts themselves and not the chest beneath!

CHOOSING THE DATE OF YOUR OPERATION

It might seem obvious but think carefully about the

date you elect to go into hospital, taking into account social events, school holidays and work. If you are a smoker or enjoy a good party or nights out with friends, plan these some time before and try to stop smoking at least six weeks prior to the operation. If they are really important to you, wait until after birthdays and Christmas festivities.

The time you need to take off work will vary according to the nature of your job. If you're in a non-strenuous role, such as administration or secretarial, you could be back at work within two weeks but if your job entails a lot of heavy lifting or stretching, you may be required to stay off for four to six weeks. Your surgeon will be the best person to advise you.

HORMONE MEDICATION

If you are taking hormone replacement therapy (HRT) or the oral contraceptive pill (OCP), you should discuss this with your surgeon at least six weeks before the operation. In general we do not stop patients taking HRT or the OCP before surgery as the risk of thrombosis in the leg veins (DVT) in patients undergoing surgery involving short general anaesthesia is very low. The significance of DVT is that a clot may go to your lung and cause a pulmonary embolus. Please ensure that this matter is fully discussed with your surgeon, preferably during your first or second consultation.

PLAN TO AVOID DETECTION

At least six weeks before the operation, you should think about how you might feel about others possibly noticing a difference in your bust size. Our advice is that if you are at all concerned about this, start wearing push-up bras such as a Wonderbra, perhaps with some extra padding. This will get them used to seeing you with a bit more upfront and hopefully, they will not bat an eyelid when the contents are real. Wearing baggy tops to disguise your figure may be another way to avoid attention.

Another method of disguising your transformation is by the use of pads (also known as 'outplants') made from specially formulated silicone that can be inserted between breast and bra. They warm to your body temperature and mould to the natural shape of the bust. Slip resistant, the pads bounce like natural breast tissue and the manufactures claim they can also be worn while swimming!

More often than not if others do notice something different about you it is not always obvious exactly what has changed. Once you are ready to face the world and go back to your normal routine, try altering the colour or style of your hair, wear a new outfit or simply swap the shade of your usual lipstick and eye shadow. Simple changes really can draw attention away from the real truth.

You should also consider the amount of time that you

will spend away from work and your social circle. In most cases, this will be a couple of weeks. A number of women have successfully used the excuse of a bad back as feasible explanation to give to children or curious family members or friends, and it's also a good excuse for you not being seen or moving with less than your usual ease and flexibility. We will usually supply a 'sick note' for your employer that mentions surgery but not the precise nature of the operation.

GENERAL HEALTH AND SMOKING

At least six weeks before the operation you should think carefully about your overall health and ensure that you are fit and healthy when you go into hospital. Maintain a proper, well-balanced diet and aim to increase your exercise levels to improve your general fitness.

If you are a smoker, aim to stop smoking altogether at least four weeks before your surgery (you may find that nicotine patches help). You should definitely cease smoking completely two weeks prior to surgery. The anaesthetist wishes to give his anaesthetic to someone who is as healthy as possible before undergoing surgery in the chest area under general anaesthetic!

Smokers are far more likely to suffer from postoperative chest problems and there is also evidence that smoking can interfere with wound healing and alter the metabolism of some drugs. Fortunately, some of the harmful effects of smoking last only a few days, so even giving up for a short time will be of great benefit. Here are some of the reasons why you will be asked to stop smoking:

- When you smoke, you breathe in carbon monoxide, which displaces oxygen from your haemoglobin, so a cigarette nervously enjoyed just before surgery can alter the oxygen-carrying capacity of your blood.
- Nicotine is a powerful drug, which causes the heart muscle to work harder and consume more oxygen. It also causes narrowing of the arteries and affects both the blood supply to your heart and to the tissues of the rest of your body. It is predominantly this mechanism that is thought to be the cause of delayed or poor wound healing.

Chest infection

When we inhale a cigarette the protective lining of the airway is suppressed so the normal ability of the lungs and the airway to clear bacteria and the dirt that we breathe in is reduced. Therefore, it is not surprising that smokers have an increased risk of chest infection after any general anaesthetic. They are much more likely to cough, leading to pain in the recently operated chest area, too. Smokers are also more inclined to bleed, partly because they cough more and raise the blood pressure.

Clotting

Smokers have 'stickier' platelets so there is a slightly increased risk of clot formation.

Capsular contracture

There is evidence to suggest smokers have a higher rate of capsule formation around the prosthesis.

CLOTHING

We suggest buying a couple of really cheap, non-underwired bras for the first week, as these will probably end up getting stained and can therefore be thrown away. It is also easier to judge your final bra size a week or so after surgery, and you can then go out and spend a bit more money on a couple of quality non-underwired sports bras. If you have followed the advice in this book so far you should already have one sports bra, the one that you took along to the initial consultation. Some women find it easier to buy a front-fastening, elasticated support bra and these are available in all major stores. Front-fastening bras and indeed tops will be more comfortable in the first few weeks than trying to pull tight-fitting clothing over your head. You will need to take one of these bras with you to hospital, where it will be fitted after your operation in theatre.

ASPIRIN AND OTHER MEDICATION

Two weeks before surgery, you should avoid taking and eating the following:

- Aspirin or aspirin-containing drugs: These thin the blood and interfere with the ability to clot, so avoid two weeks before any surgery.
- Exotic food and herbal medicines: There is some evidence to suggest that the artificial flavourings in Chinese food can weaken the blood. Our advice is to avoid excessive ingestion of Thai and Chinese food in the two weeks leading up to surgery.
- Vitamins and supplements: If you are taking vitamin E supplements, you should stop two weeks prior to surgery because excessive amounts can impair blood clotting. Also, avoid food that is high in vitamin E, including nuts, vegetable oil, potato crisps, avocados and egg yolks.

- Make sure your surgeon is fully aware of any prescribed medication that you are taking – it is wise to take these along with you to the hospital. Your surgeon should also be informed if you have allergic reactions to any drugs or dressings.

AMAZING ARNICA

One week before the operation, take a daily dose of arnica to help reduce the amount of bruising afterwards. In total, a two-week supply should be purchased so that it can be taken for a week after surgery.

As with all homeopathic medicines, arnica should be dissolved under the tongue or simply chewed, not swallowed whole and do not take with food or drink. Smoking and toothpaste should be avoided for at least thirty minutes before and after taking arnica. Also, be aware that the dose can easily be contaminated so try to avoid touching it with your fingers. Taking a stronger dose or twice the recommended amount will not have any greater effect; it is the frequency that matters. Arnica can also help with exhaustion after physical or mental effort and may well smooth postoperative recovery, as well as decrease the amount of bruising.

COLDS AND FLU

If, within two weeks of the operation you develop a sore throat and temperature or any other illness, you should inform the surgeon's clinic and obtain the necessary advice. Usually, a common cold will not seriously affect your general anaesthetic.

PREGNANCY

If you think there is a possibility that you may be pregnant, you should inform your surgeon immediately;

there are risks to the developing foetus from the drugs used for general anaesthesia.

ALCOHOL

No excessive alcohol should be consumed within the forty-eight hours prior to surgery. Alcohol is a sedative and if your brain and liver have adapted to the sedative effect, this can alter your body's response to anaesthetic drugs. You will be asked your normal alcohol consumption. This is to aid the anaesthetist as regular or heavy drinkers may require larger doses of anaesthetic to knock them out and keep them asleep.

THE NIGHT BEFORE

On the evening prior to surgery, or early on the morning of surgery, take a shower and wash your hair to ensure your whole body is cleansed. Be sure to remove any nail polish and make-up, contact lenses and jewellery (particularly metallic body piercings) while you are at home.

Leave make-up off, otherwise you will wake with it in your eyes – protective eye lubricants during the surgery make a total mess of mascara. Similarly, do not moisturise your body before the operation.

If the operation is being performed under general anaesthetic you will be asked not to eat or drink anything from midnight, the night before the operation. Sometimes, if the operation is at midday, you will be advised not to eat or drink for six hours before the operation. Many patients get nervous and this suppresses the appetite, however many more wish they had eaten more the day before as they await surgery, starving and thirsty!

Please leave any valuables at home but you may take this book, along with any light reading material that you might enjoy. You may also wish to take in an iPod with your own music; all rooms in the hospital will have a television.

Make sure that you take a loose-fitting, front-fastening top or blouse with you to wear on discharge from the hospital. It is also a good idea to bring a loose-fitting skirt or a pair of comfortable tracksuit bottoms to wear later as you may find your stomach is somewhat bloated. Air can be swallowed as part of the operation and you may experience a bit of fluid retention. We also advise that you take a pair of flat, comfortable shoes to slip on to minimise bending and straining.

GETTING TO HOSPITAL

Make sure well in advance that you know exactly how to reach the hospital and have the telephone number to hand in case you are delayed by traffic. Allow for the morning rush hour, which in London begins as early as 6.30am.

If you intend coming by car and you are not used to driving either into London or around London (or any other big city), it's a good idea to do a 'dummy run' so that your driver knows exactly where to go. Also, make sure that you have planned where to park your car (details of local car parks can be obtained from the hospital or the practice). Make arrangements for someone to drive you home because you will receive medication that makes driving yourself unsafe straight after surgery.

PREPARE FOR YOUR RETURN HOME

After surgery you will be instructed not to lift any heavy items (more than 23kg/50lb or so). It is therefore a sensible precaution, especially if you have no one at home to assist you during this time, to make some simple preparations in the week leading up to your operation. Go through your daily routine and see how many times you need to vigorously lift your arms. For example, food on high shelves should be moved lower and all loose-fitting, front-fastening tops should be on the lower shelves of your wardrobe.

Think about things that you will need to have within easy reach of your bed, such as drinks, magazines, books, the telephone and even a TV remote control. Practise putting your weight or pressure on your arms – for example, try propping yourself up in bed and notice how this affects your chest muscles. You will not want to put any excessive strain or pressure on them for the first few days because this will be painful.

PREPARATION FOR SURGERY

Think about healthy, well-balanced foods and supplements before you go into hospital and try to plan meals that are easy to prepare. It is doubtful you will want to go shopping or carry heavy shopping bags from the supermarket, or drive your car for the first few days, so stock up before surgery. Order online or pick up whatever you like to enjoy after surgery, including some lighter foods such as crackers and eggs, as well as your regular favourites.

To ensure the best possible recovery, have someone (or perhaps several people) who can all take turns to help you at home throughout the early days. This is particularly important if you have young children.

Eat a well-balanced diet. This is the optimal way of promoting the best possible recovery; it ensures the necessary vitamins, proteins and minerals are received by your body. Particular care and planning is required if you are a vegetarian or vegan. Vitamin E, which you are encouraged to avoid before your surgery, is now important for the healing process.

Along with eating a well-balanced diet, it is important to keep up your sugar levels. Sugar can help wounds heal faster as it provides glucose, a valuable food utilised in the production of heat and energy and also a tissue builder. If you are the type of person who finds it hard to give up a diet of junk food or you are used to eating ready meals, it would be wise to ask your surgeon for advice regarding mineral and vitamin supplements. However, if you follow a healthy diet, taking your regular five units of fruit or vegetables a day, then dietary supplements or multivitamins should not be required.

GETTING HOME

Ensure that you have a telephone number for both the surgeon and the hospital that can be used twenty-four hours a day in the event of an emergency following your discharge.

Make sure that you have someone to collect you from the hospital once you have undergone surgery and are ready to go home. You will not be allowed to drive and you should certainly not be travelling in taxis, trains or buses. If you have a choice of vehicle, pick one with good suspension to minimise the effect of any bumps on the journey home. Remember:

• You are not allowed to take yourself home!
• You will not be allowed to take public transport alone!
• You *must* arrange for someone to accompany you home!

This is because the pain relief medication that we prescribe can make you feel drowsy and impair your normal reactions.

PREPARATION FOR SURGERY

WHAT LOVED ONES NEED TO KNOW AND EXPECT (REQUIRED READING FOR YOUR PARTNER)

This book tries to indicate that preoperatively, a lot of time is necessary to gain the requisite information before the woman in your life makes her final decision. You must become a good listener and get used to her endless talk about her forthcoming boob job. During this time, humour, patience and support are the most important attributes.

It cannot be stressed enough just how important it is to give her your full attention and support. As with many others whose partners have undergone breast enlargement, it is not unusual to experience feelings of uncertainty as to whether or not your partner should go ahead with surgery. Most people love their other half and would not mind her staying as she is. However, many can appreciate that a person as a whole is more important and even if something were to go wrong during surgery, it would not change the way you feel about her. It is therefore important that you understand the risks associated with this type of surgery as much as your partner – after all, if it is an operation that is going to make her happier, then you should support her through it just as you would expect her to do the same if the roles were reversed.

It is important to appreciate that the first week after surgery can be difficult due to your partner's discomfort. Be prepared that after the surgery, she will experience many different emotions, unpredictable for her as well as you. She may be anxious, silent or even close to tears.

The drive to hospital should be as smooth as possible without the extra aggravation of getting lost or being late. Of course the wait before surgery may well be tense, especially after the anaesthetist has completed his/her preoperative check. At this point your partner may well feel most anxious about the general anaesthetic itself.

You may not realise how much psychological as well as physical support she will require, particularly in the first twenty-four hours at home. For some women, coming to terms with her new breasts/body shape can be as traumatic as giving birth to a child. For all women, this is the time when they need someone close to them by their side. That person is you, and you should be there for the birth of her new breasts, which will be there for life and not just for Christmas!

Some patients have a high threshold for pain and others will be lower. You will know from previous experiences what to expect in this regard. Do your best to make the journey home as smooth and pleasant as possible. A reclining seat in the car may help and pressure from the seatbelt can be alleviated with a rolled-up scarf or towel between it and her breasts.

Once home, it is probably best that your partner goes straight to bed and you sleep in different rooms initially, or on separate beds as movement may aggravate any discomfort. You should expect to do everything and anything for your partner's comfort. Soon you will notice that she becomes happier and she will improve hour by hour, any doubts swiftly disappearing from her face.

Sometimes, particularly if there is swelling, the initial view of the breasts without any dressings can be an anxious moment. A reassuring smile at this stage goes a long way. Remember, most women will not have previously undergone breast augmentation so she will be unsure of exactly what to expect and any small sign or symptom is apt to be misinterpreted as a complication. These fears and doubts will soon subside with passing time so try and mask your true feelings by reassuring your partner that there is still plenty of time for things to change and for her breasts to look and feel normal, which they will do.

At first she may be reticent to show you her new breasts, even though they might be quite hard to conceal. Soon you may find that you start to think about your partner's new breasts as much as she does.

Unfortunately, it seems that the majority of surgeons and/or clinics tend to overlook or dismiss the possibility of postoperative depression. It is better to be forewarned of the possibility of anxiety and/or depression than to be completely unprepared. If your partner does become depressed or anxious, you yourself may become upset or feel guilty in the belief that you may have helped to make this situation occur. We are just beginning to realise that a not inconsiderable number of women pass through a 'low' patch in the weeks after their augmentation. This invariably settles very quickly and seems not to have any organic basis. It may perhaps relate to a feeling of anti-climax once the long-awaited operation is finally over.

Perhaps understandably, there is a general trend among breast augmentees in the first year to experience a desire to buy and wear flattering, figure-hugging and revealing clothing. The new look provided by larger breasts is such a wonderful, much longed-for experience that many women want to enjoy and show them off as much as possible. Once her new breasts are less of a novelty, your partner will likely settle into a more conservative dress style with which she feels comfortable! If you are of a jealous disposition, you should take note of this and make allowances. Make sure you communicate with her directly rather than harbour any feelings of resentment or jealousy. Do not sulk or be moody; be proud of your partner, stand back and watch as the heads turn! You should feel encouraged in the knowledge that you helped her to achieve her desired look and the support and encouragement you provide during recovery should strengthen your relationship, bringing you closer than before the experience.

PREPARATION FOR SURGERY

You and your partner

Your partner will probably worry far more than you do, and this must not be overlooked. Women do not always realise quite how concerned their man is (men have a tendency to keep these things to themselves so as not to appear 'weak'). It is important that he understands the whole procedure of breast augmentation just as much as you do. As you embark on research and start your consultations, you will find that most of your thoughts and emotions will be centred on you and your breasts. Most partners are very supportive once they understand what it is you want. Some, however, need more convincing, while others will be very against it.

It would be unwise to go ahead without the support of your partner as it will be impossible to keep it from him: the months of research and uncertainty, plus the emotional turmoil that you will go through will all take their toll on your relationship. He needs to be convinced that what you are considering will truly make you happier and most certainly, he will be highly concerned about someone taking a surgical knife to your breast. If possible, we recommend that you encourage your partner (or a close friend or relative) to attend the consultations with you. In so doing, they can hear the surgeon explain exactly what is involved and will also be able to meet and form their own opinion regarding your choice of surgeon. They can also

141

address any concerns of their own, and may well bring up useful questions and observations that you may not have considered.

10

THE OPERATION

THE JOURNEY TO HOSPITAL

You should be aware of the time that you have been asked to arrive at the hospital and allow yourself plenty of leeway (traffic in London and other big cities can become very congested at certain times). Parking adjacent to some hospitals can also be limited. As previously suggested, do a practice run and check out the parking in advance (your hospital will be able to advise).

It is also important that you arrive in good time as any anxiety during the journey to hospital can result in your blood pressure being raised.

As previously mentioned, you should wear no make-up. Also, you should not oil your body, or use lotions or potions; these will interfere with the marking process.

HOSPITAL ADMISSION

If your operation is in the morning, you should not eat after midnight the day before (whatever the time of your operation, you should abstain from food for six hours in advance). At the hospital, you will be asked to sign some consent and patient information forms before you are admitted.

Once on the ward, you will find the rooms a little like hotel accommodation, each one equipped with a television and an en-suite bathroom.

You will be asked to change into a gown and provided with paper underwear and TED (Thrombo-Embolic Deterrent) stockings (to prevent deep vein thrombosis). At this point, remove any metallic jewellery or body piercings (this prevents any electrical contact on the operating table, causing burns).

You will then be visited by your anaesthetist; he/she will already be aware of your medical record but will again go through your past medical history and ask you about previous anaesthetics, plus any allergies or significant medical conditions you may have and also discuss your teeth. This is also the time to discuss pain control and nausea prevention.

You are then seen by your surgeon, who will confirm the operation, size and type of prosthesis and the position of the pockets. He/she will sign the hospital consent form with you. This is a standard form and includes the name of the proposed operation, what is to be achieved by that operation and any possible complications. You will be asked to sign the form to confirm that you understand and have been given the opportunity to ask questions; also that you have read and studied the patient information leaflets.

The surgeon will then mark out your chest. He/she will remind you of any asymmetry, if marked. Do not be alarmed by the lines, which do not signify where the incisions are to be made; they are merely a guide for the surgeon as to the dissection of the pocket in which the prosthesis will be positioned. You should wear your chosen bra the right way round and low down like a belt. This makes it much easier to put on when you are asleep.

THEATRE
You will be then escorted down to theatre, usually walking with the nurse. No premedication drugs are given these days. In rare instances a premedication may be administered, in which case you will be taken to theatre on a trolley.

THE ANAESTHETIC
Most anaesthetics are given intravenously, i.e. the

wrist is squeezed and a small needle placed in the back of the hand (you will only feel 'a little scratch'). Needle-phobic patients are anaesthetised by placing a mask over the face and breathing in gas. A cannula (small plastic tube) will be inserted in a vein once you are asleep to allow anaesthetic, fluids and antibiotics to be given.

THE OPERATING THEATRE

Once asleep, you will then be taken from the anaesthetic room into the operating theatre, where you will be positioned on the operating table. As well as the anti-embolus (TED) stockings, special boots will be placed on the calf muscles to pump the blood away from your legs at regular intervals.

The chest wall will now be infiltrated with a mixture of Marcaine (a long-acting local anaesthetic) and Adrenaline (to decrease bleeding and bruising). This is injected into the subcutaneous tissues (between the skin and the muscle) of the chest wall. The chest wall is then painted with an antiseptic. In most cases, this is an iodine solution unless you have previously mentioned any allergy to iodine; this accounts for the yellow colour your skin will probably have after surgery. Your nipples will be covered with a sterile plastic film because bacteria reside in the ducts opening out onto the nipple and cannot be sterilised.

The surgeon will then formally mark out your

breast, allowing for asymmetry, the size of the prosthesis and in particular the area of the base of the prosthesis; also, how far towards the mid-line and the side of the chest the pocket will extend. He/ she will then use a ruler to measure the exact length of the incision and its exact position in relation to the other side. The incision is usually 4–5cm (1.5–2in) long and lies at the inferior aspect of the base of the prosthesis, which is usually close to the inframammary groove.

Smaller incisions are suggested by some surgeons claiming greater expertise and occasionally very small incisions if saline-filled prostheses are being used, especially when inserted from some distant point on the anatomy, such as the belly button.

There is some evidence that excessive manipulation of silicone gel prostheses, especially the high cohesive ones, through a very small incision can lead to the silicone gel fracturing and possibly also damaging the shell. We strongly recommend a decent-sized incision be used to avoid over-manipulation of the implant and allow atraumatic dissection of the pocket (delicate dissection with no tearing). In any case, when fully matured your scar should sit in the crease and be unnoticeable, except with close inspection.

The pocket for the prosthesis is then dissected. This is done with electrical cauterisation, which allows even the smallest of blood vessels to be coagulated.

The surgical plane underneath the pectoralis major muscle is almost bloodless and therefore there is minimal trauma. Everyone's muscle is a little different in terms of the fine detail of the anatomy. For instance, sometimes more muscle has to be dissected (i.e. divided towards the breastbone), but we caution against over-dissection to try and create a midline cleavage as the effect of the muscle covering the prosthesis can be lost.

Inferiorly, the muscle may be divided, particularly when a biplanar pocket is being developed for a droopy breast. Use of anatomical implants makes us dissect small pockets that need to be the exact size for the prosthesis as a large pocket will allow the prosthesis to move about and there have been reported cases of the prosthesis rotating and even flipping over with disastrous results from the point of view of trying to achieve a natural shape.

When both pockets have been dissected, they are irrigated with a solution of antibiotics. The prostheses are then inserted into the pockets in an extremely sterile way whereby they are only touched by the surgeon. Following this, the patient is then sat up on the operating table so that the position of the prosthesis and the symmetry can be compared on both sides. Once the surgeon is happy, the wounds are sutured in three layers using dissolving sutures so there is no need for stitches to be removed at a later date. At this point the long-acting painkiller Marcaine and further antibiotic solution will be inserted into the pocket. The operation is complete after cleaning the breast – when all the bleeding has been controlled and the pocket has been washed out with the antibiotic cocktail. A waterproof dressing is applied to the surgical incision, which is then covered with tape to allow early postoperative showering. A strap is applied across the top of the breast to prevent the implants from riding up and a sports bra usually applied.

We believe the ABBA Technique has been proven to give the best results with regard to the outcome of capsular contracture. This involves:

- An inframammary incision
- A submuscular pocket
- Minimal traumatic dissection technique
- Perfect haemostasis (arrest of bleeding)
- Most importantly, use of mixed antibiotic solutions provide a sterile operative procedure
- Following surgery, antibiotics must be taken for five days.

The result of all this extra care and attention is that the operation takes a little longer. For the patient, speed should not be an issue. However, it can be an issue for some larger clinics, who try to squeeze in as many cases each day, like a factory production line. Some perform as many as fourteen breast augmentations in a day and you would perhaps not wish to be number thirteen! Look for a surgeon who, while experienced and dexterous, can be relied on to allow sufficient time for a meticulous surgical technique with regard to the dissection of the pocket into which the prosthesis will be placed.

Again, the number of cases the surgeon has done should not be a major issue. What is the point of a surgeon having completed thousands of breast augmentations if he/she has no accurate record of the complications, his/her own true capsular contracture rate, his/her re-operation rate or published his/her work on breast augmentation in a peer-reviewed journal?

RECOVERY

The anaesthetist will have prepared your anaesthetic so that as the surgeon completes the dressing, you will wake up. With a cough, the tube in your mouth will be removed and you will be amazed at how alert some patients are – feeling they have just taken a 'power nap'. Most have little pain at this time.

With an oxygen mask in position, you will be taken on a trolley to be formally received in the recovery unit. There, you will be assigned an individual specialist nurse to regularly monitor your pulse, blood pressure, breathing and pain levels. Once your recovery is stable, the anaesthetist will check that you are continuing to recover well and usually within half an hour you will be transferred back to the ward, where your recovery will be further monitored.

11

POSTOPERATIVE
RECOVERY

The better your surgeon performs and the more carefully you follow instructions, the more rapidly you will recover from your operation. Full normal activity in three days or less is possible, although you will not be partying!

Recovering from breast augmentation is different to preparing for it. Throughout the preparation there are many ways to actively change the course of events. During recovery your body will automatically do most of the work, provided you do not expect everything to happen quickly or mess with the autopilot. If you understand what is normal, what to expect and some of the reasons behind the do's and don'ts, your recovery process will be much smoother. Small things can make a big difference and for the first week or so, front-fastening bras and loose-fitting clothing will be more comfortable.

RECOVERY IS VARIABLE

What you can do to improve your recovery depends on the surgeon but how you feel varies from patient to patient. From one woman to another, the body and breast tissues are different; the tighter your breast skin envelope and the more surgical manipulation required, the more tightness and tenderness you can expect. Everyone can expect some tightness and tenderness but the amount varies from patient to patient. Hence, if you had children prior to your breast augmentation, the tissues will have been stretched naturally. Therefore, the feeling of tightness will be less than if your skin and breast is very tight and has never previously been stretched or expanded.

Some patients are more tolerant of discomfort than others and are said to have a higher pain threshold. Despite discomfort, some are better able to get moving after surgery and some will follow instructions better than others. Some are more motivated to a quick recovery than others; some are optimistic and others take a more pessimistic view, so 'normal' is as varied as in other areas of life.

Your individual pain tolerance, motivation and ability to follow instructions all affect your recovery. The same is true of your mental state: adopt a positive attitude and you will recover sooner.

SURGEON VARIATIONS

A surgeon cannot change what you bring him/her to work with, but how he/she works with what you bring can affect your recovery. The less surgical trauma the surgeon causes to your tissues, the easier and shorter your recovery will be. For instance, if your tissues are thin and submuscular placement of the implants was undertaken, you will have more tenderness, but this is short-term inconvenience in return for the long-term protection and gains in terms of feeling the prosthesis and capsular contracture. If your surgeon uses blunt dissection techniques, you can expect more tenderness and bruising, with the possible inconvenience of drains – plastic tubes inserted into wounds to drain blood and fluid, which are connected to plastic bags or bottles.

The easier your surgeon expects your recovery to be, the shorter the list of postoperative instructions. And the more he/she can do in the operating theatre, the less you will be burdened with after surgery. Surgeons' postoperative instructions vary widely, so follow your own surgeon's advice very carefully: he/she knows what has been done during the operation and therefore what needs to be done postoperatively. Do not follow a friend's postoperative instructions.

If your surgeon is giving instructions that sound a lot

simpler than you have heard from a friend, be grateful: he/she has probably done a lot more in the operating theatre and has simply made life easier for you. On the other hand, if your surgeon tells you not to do things, there are usually good reasons for this so always follow the instructions.

YOUR SURGEON'S STAFF

Remember, your surgeon's team should be an extension of him/her. Their goal should be to help you get better sooner and to reassure you. When you ring the surgeon's office, listen carefully to any questions and instructions that you are given. The information you give them and the way you convey it will help the staff make the best recommendations to speed your recovery. Some surgeons have better staff than others. If you are left in doubt about anything after speaking to the staff, ask to speak directly with your surgeon or make an appointment to see him/her.

PAIN MEDICATION

Pain medication is a double-edged sword so the less you need, the better. It is necessary for the relief of pain, but can interfere with recovery. The stronger the medication, the more relief or discomfort it will provide, but more adverse effects are also possible and the worst of these are drowsiness, nausea and constipation.

The best thing is to get moving and to take only as

much painkiller as you need. Here, the trick is to use enough pain medication to deal with the discomfort at first and as soon as you get moving, things will get better and you will need fewer painkillers. If you do not get moving, your recovery will definitely take longer and be more difficult. Getting moving does not mean aerobic exercise – just resume normal activities.

Always line your stomach with milk or food before taking pain medication, to protect your stomach from certain types of painkiller that may cause ulcers.

Using today's surgical techniques you should not need any pain medication stronger than codeine or a codeine-equivalent drug. Most patients take codeine or a codeine-equivalent medication for the first forty-eight to seventy-two hours and then switch to paracetamol.

If you know what to expect and what is normal, you will be less frightened or concerned. Recovery is so much easier if you arm yourself with knowledge. Here is a checklist of everything that is normal following surgery, so expect it and continue to expect it, for at least six weeks after surgery.

- They do not match – my breasts are different sizes and shapes
- They are too high/too low/too big/too tight/too swollen/too firm
- I hear sloshing inside my breasts
- My breasts do not move
- They are numb, too sensitive, or feel funny

- I cannot lie on them because they feel like grapefruits.

Remember, the best breasts never match: your genes could not make them match and neither can your surgeon. Early on after surgery you will always have more swelling on one side than the other, maybe adding to the difference; this is normal. Your breasts are supposed to feel too big, too firm, too swollen and too tight or too weird. Remember, yesterday you did not have this much inside your breast. It takes time for your skin envelope to adapt and stretch.

After surgery, with or without drains, you will produce a little fluid inside the pocket around your implant. Combined with a small amount of air that stays in the pocket from surgery, this fluid can produce a sloshing sound that you may or may not hear for a week or two after surgery. Do not worry: your body will absorb the excess air and fluid. Sometimes the air gets trapped in the tissues and produces a bubblewrap effect. This surgical emphysema, as it is called, will soon spontaneously disappear. The larger the implants, the tighter the skin envelop and the more stretch on the implant, the more pressure on surrounding structures, including nerves.

Nerves respond in two to three ways: they can go numb, concuss, become more sensitive or send odd sensations back to your brain. Regardless of surgical technique, sensory changes are therefore variable and very unpredictable. They can also take a long time to resolve, as much as two years, although most patients recover sensation far more quickly than this and some experience no problems at all. Any nipple discomfort can be alleviated by putting clingfilm (plastic wrap) over them to avoid rubbing against your clothing.

WHAT IS ABNORMAL?

If you develop any of the following symptoms, you should contact your surgeon immediately:

- A temperature higher than a 39°C (102°F) or fever with chills
- One breast that is much larger than the other
- One breast that appears much more bruised than the other
- Noticeable redness and tenderness in any area of the breast
- Any drainage from your incision after three days
- Any unusual discomfort or breathing problems
- Anything to cause you great concern and that you yourself feel is abnormal.

Remember, do not suffer alone: we are there to help.

DAY CASES/GOING HOME

When you leave the hospital as a day case, you may well feel a bit drowsy but comfortable. This is because of all the medication you have been given. When you get home, make yourself comfortable on a chair or bed, drink some water and eat a light meal – nothing too heavy or rich, something gentle on your stomach. Limit tea and coffee and avoid alcohol, as it is dehydrating and may interact with antibiotics. We suggest that you take a strong painkiller after eating and expect to relax and feel drowsy as a result of this (you will probably doze on and off). We recommend that you have a competent adult staying with you for 24 hours after a general anaesthetic.

You will already have raised your arms above your head before leaving the hospital in order to get your clothes on but once home, do this at least three times before going to sleep. Regular gentle arm movements are important to prevent stiffness. At first just lift them until they are level with your shoulders. If you feel tightness but no pain, go ahead and lift them above your head. Lower and repeat twice more. Between sleep, repeat this entire sequence as best you can every three hours. You will be amazed at how much easier the rest of your recovery will be.

When you feel really hungry and have no nausea, have a small meal (usually breakfast the next day). Once you have some food inside you, take a stronger painkiller and enjoy your rest. If you wake up during the night, rearrange yourself to get comfortable and try to go back to sleep. Sometimes hugging a pillow to your chest can make you feel better.

When you wake up in the morning, you will feel stiff but this is perfectly normal. You would not believe how much better you will feel after getting your arms moving. Expect to feel tightness, but that is also normal – you will not damage anything by lifting your arms above your head. Now it all depends on you and how you are feeling. If you feel like a short walk outside, then do it but if you prefer to sit around at home and relax, do that. The important thing is to keep moving and to keep exercising your arms.

Within forty-eight hours, it should not be necessary to take the strong painkillers you will have been given and now you can take the less powerful painkillers, as and when required (they do not need to be taken at regular intervals throughout the day). It may be a good idea to continue to use the stronger painkillers at bedtime for better sleep. Do be careful of constipation, though: this can occur if you take too many painkillers and for too long. You should not be in a lot of pain; pain is the body's warning system so if you are experiencing severe pain, you should be calling your surgeon for advice.

Among surgeons, there is some disagreement as to what is the best painkiller. Non-steroidal anti-inflammatory drugs (NSAIDs) can interfere with platelet function (the elements of the bloodstream that contribute to blood clotting) and therefore may affect bleeding. However, this is more theoretical than practical.

Because wounds take forty-eight hours to become waterproof, the first days you should sit in a shallow bath and keep your dressings dry. After a few days, however, you may take a shower and wash your hair. However, do not rub the dressings too hard; simply pat them dry with a towel.

As soon as you feel like picking up normal weight objects or your small children (no more than 23kg/50lb), do so. Most of our patients with young families are able to pick them up a day or two after surgery. Of course it all depends on the size of child, but you will not damage anything. Just avoid heavy objects and straining.

Be sure to drink plenty of liquids and resume your normal healthy diet as soon as possible. As soon as you can, cease the strong prescription pain medications (Tramadol, Co-proxamol, Co-codamol, Tylex and the like), which cause constipation, nausea and a general feeling of tiredness and light-headedness.

Do not be surprised if you feel bloated after surgery: you received fluids during your operation and you will naturally accumulate some swelling around the breasts and chest. This swelling gravitates downwards and you will begin to feel your waist is getting bigger, but do not panic: this will resolve itself. You will also find that you pass water more often as your kidneys work at removing the extra fluid.

The first two days after surgery are filled with the

most aggravation and discomfort. After two days, start thinking about the next three weeks. Aim to return to most of your normal activities as soon as possible – of course, this may be governed by things like work and childcare – and just plan your days to allow for some rest if you get tired.

THE FIRST THREE WEEKS

Listen to your body when it comes to full activity. If something is too stressful, stop and try again tomorrow – your body will tell you what you need to know. Just listen. That does not mean stopping everything, but if something really hurts, stop. Try again later.

As to your mental state, a short period of low mood or depression is not uncommon and increasingly recognised by surgeons. Whether it is some form of anaesthetic 'hangover' or simply the anti-climax of the surgery being over after what for some people has been many years of waiting, is unknown but it should settle of its own accord in a short time. Of course, you should contact your GP if any depression persists.

When you are comfortable, sex is fine. You would probably not feel overly amorous if a partner put too much pressure on your breasts after the first few days, but there are ways around that. 'Look good, feel bad' takes on a whole new meaning when your breasts feel better. Your significant other may require some coaching and understanding at first. By all means be creative, but save the Olympic-level sex for a few weeks down the road!

DRIVING A CAR

Again, there is no strict specific date and some patients will drive an automatic car freely three days after surgery. Others may take up to two weeks to feel comfortable enough to drive a heavy manual car. There is no reason, however, why you cannot get back to driving a car within a few days after surgery, but make it easier on yourself by placing a rolled scarf or soft towel between your new breasts and beneath the seatbelt for comfort.

WEARING A BRA

It's totally up to you but if you feel more comfortable in a bra (perhaps to create a certain look), wear one. We suggest a supportive sports bra for the first six weeks. If you are more comfortable without a bra, do not wear one. Despite anything you might hear, a bra should not affect the results of your surgery. We understand that you know better than anyone else what makes you feel comfortable and therefore we give you the choice. Be aware, though that your breasts undergo big changes throughout the first few weeks so finding the best one takes patience.

We advise you not to wear an underwired bra until six weeks after the operation and then only on high days or holidays. This is because the weakest part of the repair is under the breast and therefore it seems reasonable not to apply too much pressure to this area, which wires technically can. As already stated, whether or not you wear a bra in the recovery period is up to you, but a supportive sports bra gives comfort and reassurance to a lot of patients.

TIME HEALS

By the end of three weeks, most of the worst discomfort and aggravation will be over but your breasts will still not feel as if they belong to you. Start thinking three months after the first three weeks.

After the first three weeks, the skin begins to relax and this is something that you will gradually notice. Remember, constantly looking in the mirror never made anyone heal quicker! As the skin relaxes, the excessive upper fullness begins to decrease provided you have not selected an excessively large implant for your tissues. The implants are not really dropping, what is really happening is that the lower skin is stretching. Also, the swelling from the upper part of the breasts migrates down the body so as the upper fullness decreases you may feel your breasts are becoming smaller. This is not the case, although you might think so because most of the time you yourself will be looking at them! Check your side view in a mirror and you will notice a gradual appearance of fullness in the lower breast. This progression happens in every augmentation: expect it and do not worry. The sequence in Figs.8a–d show how long this can take.

Suddenly shopping is a lot more fun and although your breasts will continue to change during the first three months, it is a whole new experience to wear anything you want and look fabulous. Different patients feel comfortable shopping at different times but when you feel like it, do it. Towards the end of the three-month period, you will begin to notice your breasts less and one day all of a sudden you will not be aware of them at all. As if by magic, they will have become part of you.

ANTIBIOTICS

On leaving the hospital, you will be given a course of antibiotics that will last for five days. It is important that you take them at regular intervals and not on an empty stomach. Should you develop any adverse symptoms (in particular, diarrhoea or an upset stomach), get in touch with your surgeon's office.

AVOID ASPIRIN

Refrain from taking aspirin as a painkiller for at least a week after surgery and if you accidentally take any medication containing aspirin, you should inform your surgeon. Always follow their advice.

BRUISING

You may notice small areas of bruising, although regular doses of arnica for a week after surgery should reduce this to a minimum. When bruising occurs this indicates that some blood from the operation has escaped into the tissues and, like water, flows downhill. Bruising contained within the muscles will not be evident, but may cause pain in much the same way as a footballer's dead leg. Of course it is painful and does limit movement but it's also an essential part of the healing process and as we have already said, at this stage it's important to keep moving.

SENSITIVITY AND NUMBNESS

At first the nipples may be extremely sensitive, yet underneath the breasts can be quite numb. These changes in sensitivity can vary throughout the recovery period for up to two years: some patients find the increased sensitivity a great problem while others find an increase in sensitivity more of a pleasure than a discomfort. One thing you cannot predict is the increase or loss of sensitivity in the breasts. Eighty-seven per cent of women participating in a survey had varying degrees of numbness or increased sensitivity and this will vary from one side to the other.

As previously suggested, if you do experience increased sensitivity in your nipples, a good tip is to cover them with clingfilm (plastic wrap) to avoid them rubbing against your clothing.

NO SMOKING

You should continue to refrain from smoking for at least two weeks after surgery. Smoking will impair your circulation and interfere with the healing process; it also makes you more likely to experience a haematoma (a collection of blood which can require further surgery) and there is now good evidence to suggest that capsular contracture rates are higher in smokers than non-smokers. If you managed to stop smoking prior to surgery, now is perhaps a good time to stop completely (help and advice is available from your GP).

ABSTAIN FROM ALCOHOL

Following surgery, some women have been advised to avoid alcohol for as much as two weeks. As with all things in life, moderation is best. Be aware that alcohol and some painkillers can summate and therefore you should be extremely cautious and not imbibe alcohol when you are on the strong painkillers.

USE LOTS OF MOISTURISER

Applying moisturiser to your chest helps prevent the skin from becoming dry. There is no evidence that massaging your breasts will prevent capsular contracture, though. However, it is a good idea to gently massage the area so that you become aware of your breasts and gain more confidence in them. Massage will help your scars to mature, but begin only after three to four weeks, using a vitamin E cream.

CARING FOR YOUR SCARS

Your incisions will seal themselves rapidly and are effectively watertight after forty-eight hours, so you may shower then. Do not bathe or swim yet, though, as they are not completely waterproof. You will first catch sight of your scars on removal of the dressings at one week. Be prepared for them to be redder in colour, more obvious and raised over the next few weeks; this is entirely normal and part of the body's healing process, so do not be alarmed. We know that the worst time for a scar is usually between six and twelve weeks when most active. After this time it will start to settle down and massage seems to help. We recommend twice daily for ten to fifteen minutes. The cream itself is probably unimportant, but there is some suggestion that those containing vitamin E may assist with scar maturation. You may use firm pressure after the first three to four weeks.

THE SUN AND ULTRAVIOLET LIGHT (UV)

Fresh scars are less able to withstand the damaging effects of UV radiation and will react more readily to the sun, so ensure that you keep them covered for the first year. Thereafter, you may expose them in order to pick up some colour and help disguise them.

POSTOPERATIVE DEPRESSION

Be patient: naturally, the recovery period will seem to drag on. Similarly to going on a diet, you may begin to wonder whether you will ever feel normal again – first you notice drastic changes, but then hit a plateau. Wait patiently for the end result. Like a rose, your breast needs time to bloom. It is exactly the same as children whose growth you cannot perceive if you see them every day. That's why surgeons are almost obsessed with photographs and we have lost count of the stunned expressions and disbelief written all over the faces of patients when they realise just how much change has occurred after being shown their preoperative photographs.

If you have any anxieties about your recovery, do not suffer in silence. Ask questions of your surgeon or his staff and never feel that you are being a nuisance. Most surgeons will have a practice nurse with many years of experience and he/she should be able to help with any non-emergency enquiries. It is easy for patients to feel isolated during recovery and some feel their aftercare was lacking or inadequate. Through reading this book you have placed yourself at a distinct advantage, ensuring that you receive nothing but the best possible advice, information and counselling, before and after surgery.

POSTOPERATIVE RECOVERY

There is something magic about three months. Around this time most of our patients feel that the implants have become part of their body – they stop referring to them as implants and start talking about 'my breasts'. The reason for this time period is because your tissues require about three months to return to their normal state.

THE MOST IMPORTANT DO'S:

- Do follow your surgeon's instructions
- Do stay hydrated – drink plenty of fluids
- Eat and eat well
- Resume normal activity as soon as possible
- Expect to be frustrated that your tissues do not change according to your schedule
- Also, expect to be too big, too high and too tight
- For three to six weeks, expect differences and constant change in the size and shape of your breasts. Get out of the house and do something to divert your mind
- Remember, staring at your breasts in a mirror won't reduce swelling and tightness
- If anything seems wrong, check your instructions and if in doubt, do not hesitate to call your surgeon.

THE MOST IMPORTANT DON'TS

- Avoid taking any pain medication on an empty stomach

- Also avoid any type of aerobic or other activity that creates a significant increase in your pulse rate for two weeks
- Walking is okay, fast walking is not
- Sex is okay, Olympic-style is off-limits!
- Do not lift heavy objects over 23kg (50lb) or strain hard for two weeks
- Avoid taking too many painkillers. This will cause constipation and can make you feel unwell. Always follow your surgeon's advice and avoid whatever he/she tells you to avoid.

THE BOTTOM LINE

- Listen to your surgeon's advice and follow it
- Be positive and active
- Aim for an early return to activity and normal daily life
- Enjoy your new breasts!

12

MASTOPEXY AUGMENTATION

Also known as 'augmentation mastopexy', this is the name given to surgery that combines breast augmentation (to increase volume) with mastopexy (to uplift, reduce the excess tissue of a stretched and droopy envelope, and elevate the nipple-areola complex/NAC closer to its rightful level).

A mastopexy is not always required to deal with ptosis (droop) and a biplanar BA may be used in mild (grade I) or moderate (grade II) degrees. While biplanar BA can certainly improve the volume deficit, it has only a limited effect on elevating the NAC and is not possible in all cases. One particular problem with using a prosthesis to effect uplift is that a larger implant than ideal is required to fill out the empty bag of skin as this condition frequently results from a pregnancy where the breasts became very enlarged or after significant weight loss.

If your surgeon considers that you will not obtain a satisfactory result from either routine breast augmentation or a biplanar breast augmentation, then you will be advised to undergo a mastopexy procedure, together with breast augmentation.

The indications for mastopexy augmention include:

- Third-degree ptosis of the breast (where the NAC lies below the inframammary fold and at the lowest part of the breast). The greater part of the breast is very low on the chest wall, sometimes even abutting onto the anterior abdominal wall. If a prosthesis is positioned in the usual place on the chest, most of the breast will lie below it and the result will be a drooping of the main substance over the breast over the prosthesis – the 'double bubble' deformity.
- Patients who have previously had very large implants inserted and wish to have smaller ones and where the overlying skin tissue cover has become very thin.
- Those who previously had large breasts and have achieved significant weight loss.
- Patients with previous breast augmentation who have developed capsule formation, particularly

with drooping – the so-called 'rock in a sock' deformity.

- May be part of reconstruction of the breast after a subcutaneous or skin sparing mastectomy.

Like many other decisions in breast surgery, augmentation mastopexy is a trade-off. It allows a patient whose breasts are droopy and empty, who would otherwise be unsuitable for breast augmentation, to have her breasts enlarged at the expense of more extensive scars. Here, it is worth emphasising that scars are an individual healing characteristic. Just because your friend has good scars or you yourself have good scarring on other parts of your body does not guarantee that you will make good scars on your breasts. If you are self-conscious about your breasts then you may well be self-conscious about your breasts with scars, even though they will be of a different shape and size (that is, fuller and higher on your chest).

Scars can vary with the type of mastopexy performed. All mastopexies involve a scar around the nipple areolar complex. Essentially, additional scars are required to remove the excess skin in the lower part of the breast. These may involve only a vertical scar running downwards from the 6 o'clock position on the NAC scar to the inframammary fold – the vertical scar mastopexy. If there is a large amount of skin to be removed, then a further scar running horizontally in the

IMF itself will be required. This is an 'Anchor Scar' (also known as a 'Wise Pattern').

Sometimes the skin tone is very good and a simple vertical scar mastopexy can be performed, which will not require the transverse scar in the inframammary groove. This is a great advantage because it is frequently the inframammary scar that produces problems. Towards the mid-line of the chest, the scar can show in low décolletage and towards the armpit, the scar can often spread.

To try and overcome the extent of scars a different procedure (so-called 'doughnut' mastopexy) has been popularised, particularly in South America. This involves a scar simply around the outside of the areola. Though seductive, it can lead to problems of bunching of the skin as it is drawn in around the reduced size of the nipple areola diameter and if there is a lot of tension the scars can stretch and spread.

Compromise is of the essence when deciding to have a mastopexy augment and indeed in accepting the type of mastopexy that will be performed with regard to the extent of scarring. Patients who have very thin skin or thin soft tissue cover with stretch marks (i.e. poor skin tone) often require more extensive scars, as described in the anchor scar arrangement.

COMPLICATIONS

The complications of mastopexy augmentation include the following:

Scarring

These scars have been described above and will be red for about three to six months. Although slowly fading, they will always be visible. They can be of good quality where skin tension is low, but in patients who demand large volume changes with a small chest, the scars can stretch and be unsightly.

Nipple Necrosis

The nipple needs to be elevated into a new position higher on the breast. If only about 2–3cm (0.7–1.2in), the nipple can be safely lifted onto the underlying breast tissue. This is the safest way of lifting the nipple and you are less likely to lose sensation. When the nipple areolar complex has to be raised more than about 5cm (2in), it must be lifted up on a tongue of breast tissue and therefore the blood and nerve supply are more precarious. Occasionally (about one in 100 cases), the blood supply may not be sufficient to support the relocated NAC and all, or part of it may die. This is more common in smokers, diabetics or patients with cardiovascular disease, or in those who wish to have very large augmentations, with high tension on the skin closure. Complete loss is rare and usually all that is required for partial losses are patience and good wound care. The scar tends to be slightly thicker and more obvious, though.

Nipple sensation
Feeling is also likely to be reduced after surgery.

Fat Necrosis
It is easy to see when more surgery is done to the breast, and in particular areas of the breasts are divided and sutures placed in the breast tissue to lift the nipple up, how small areas of the breast tissue can die. This is known as 'fat necrosis' and while benign, may result in a lump in the breast. This usually resolves itself over two to three months without any specific treatment. If there is a large area of fat necrosis then the breast may become red with a discharge from the suture line, sparking fears that the breast is infected. However, if it is pure fat necrosis then this will often settle without any specific long-term effects.

Skin Necrosis
Again, this is more common in smokers and diabetics. It occurs when the skin closure is tight, either because too large a prosthesis is being inserted or too much skin has been excised and the skin closure is tight. Skin necrosis rarely requires any specific treatment except when sufficient to reveal the underlying prosthesis, which may then become infected and extrude. This is why many surgeons prefer to place the prosthesis under the muscle in mastopexy.

Haematoma

Bleeding is more common in mastopexy augmentation than straightforward breast augmentation, but still a rare complication. Many surgeons insert drains to try and overcome this complication, but there is some evidence that drains may increase infection and capsular contraction.

Infection

Again more common than for standard breast augmentation, usually infection results from a skin-healing problem that may end up in the prosthesis being lost.

Malposition

Probably the most common complication of mastopexy augmentation is malposition of the prosthesis. All patients should be warned that the technical judgement of trying to produce symmetry in a mastopexy augment is difficult, despite the fact that the patient is sitting up during the operation to try and confirm symmetry. The fact that after this surgery there is a difference in the height of the two breasts requiring an adjustment is not considered malpractice, provided the patient has been advised before surgery takes place that this is a possibility and does not reflect incompetence on the surgeon's part. All surgeons agree that obtaining symmetry is impossible. Some will only do this operation as a two-stage procedure because they have difficulty in achieving symmetry of the nipple areolar complexes, so the mastopexy is done as a first stage and breast augmentation as a second stage.

Occasionally patients who are reluctant to accept the scars of a mastopexy are prepared to undergo a breast augmentation using the biplanar technique and if sufficient NAC elevation is not obtained, will then elect to undergo secondary mastopexy at a later stage. This may also be the decision of patients who undergo augmentation and then have a subsequent pregnancy or lose a lot of weight and have an acceptable result from breast augmentation apart from the fact that the nipple areolar complexes have drooped over high breast prosthesis.

THE OPERATIVE PROCEDURE

In many ways, the operative procedure is similar to a breast reduction:

1. Informed consent is required
2. The operative plan is made and discussed. This includes:
   - The prosthesis pocket – either in front of or under the pectoralis major muscle
   - How the nipple areolar complex will be raised on the chest wall, i.e. will it be on a glandular pedicle or on a pedicle of breast tissue?

- The type of skin excision to be undertaken and therefore the resulting extent of scarring.
- (All of this should be decided before surgery is undertaken.)
3. Sizing: Also an issue, sizing can be determined by the standard methods of using sizers and fitting them inside a sports bra with the desired cup size, or via 3D photography and computer morphing.

You will be admitted to hospital in the normal way and usually this operation is undertaken with an overnight stay. As part of the admission procedure you will be admitted, seen and assessed by the anaesthetist. You will sign a consent form and your breasts will be marked out and measured in a standard way.

The principal markings will be:

- To measure and choose the position of the new nipple areolar complex (NAC).
- To mark the inframammary fold.

Some surgeons do not choose the new position of the NAC until the implant has been inserted and do this with you in the operating theatre, asleep and sitting up.

The standard procedure is to then perform the breast augmentation. Usually this is undertaken through a standard incision in the inframammary fold, but if no scar is anticipated in this area, it will be done through the vertical incision scar. For many surgeons a submuscular pocket is dissected and the prosthesis positioned into this pocket. Some surgeons favour a pocket in front of the muscle, but the risk of extrusion is higher if there is skin breakdown post-operatively. Once the augmentation has been successfully undertaken, the patient is sat up on the operating table. The positions of the intended nipple areolar complexes are either confirmed or estimated, as is the amount of skin to be excised.

The first part of the mastopexy is to lift the nipple-areolar complex on its pedicle into its new position. This involves cutting a circle of skin higher on the chest at the point of estimation and the incision made around the nipple-areolar complex, the skin excised between the two positions and the nipple elevated.

The gland of the breast is then repositioned, usually by making a cone that helps support the elevated nipple-areolar complex and lifts the whole breast higher onto the chest wall. Following this the skin is excised, as previously estimated. Wound closure usually employs a buried absorbable stitch to close the skin.

RECOVERY

Usually this procedure is undertaken with an overnight stay in hospital. If drains are inserted, these are removed before departure the following day if drainage volumes are acceptable. Usually the breast is supported with a brassière made out of Elastoplast, with the patient's own bra over the top.

Recovery is essentially the same as for standard breast augmentation – with one important exception. Immediately after the operation and during the ensuing hours, the nursing staff will regularly assess the blood supply to the nipple by looking and pressing it regularly.

With much larger incisions, wound healing may take longer and the need to have dressings changed beyond two weeks may be necessary, especially at the T-scars (at the junctions of NAC and IMF and vertical scars), where tension is greatest. By six weeks all wounds are generally healed and breast swelling will be settling to reveal reasonable and acceptable symmetry.

Perfect symmetry is never achievable, however in most cases a compromise is acceptable. Adjustments to the position of implants may be required. This should not be considered a negligent complication and can occur in the best of hands.

THE BOTTOM LINE

Complications of mastopexy augmentation are obviously more common than in straightforward breast augmentation. The risks are increased in smokers, patients with hypertension, Diabetes mellitus and where it is the patient's choice to have a very large prosthesis inserted, resulting in a high degree of skin tension. Notwithstanding this, serious complications are rare.

13

MAINTENANCE

Maintenance really means the long-term future care following a successful breast augmentation. Given that breast implants are man-made and should not be considered lifetime devices, it is likely to occur in all such cases of women who live long enough.

Other than device failure, there are a number of complications that may require further surgery without necessarily affecting the long-term cosmetic outcome. Moreover, the breast is an active organ, whose size, shape and dimensions change throughout life and particularly after pregnancy and breastfeeding, so expect some form of maintenance surgery at some point. Listed below are the common concerns.

Prosthesis of the wrong size or unacceptable asymmetry

All patients will say they are very happy with the outcome of their breast augmentation, but wish that they had chosen a prosthesis that was a little bigger. This is why preoperative photographs are so important because it is easy to forget what one looked like. As we become better at sizing and understanding that the trial implant always ends up appearing a little smaller when inside the body, this should become less of a problem. This is where 3D imaging comes into its own.

There are patients who feel they are too small and very occasionally, too big. Obviously the only way that this can be corrected is by reoperation and using differently sized prosthesis.

Rupture of the prosthesis

It is often very difficult for a patient to realise that their prosthesis has ruptured. Occasionally, severe trauma such as a road traffic accident and blunt chest trauma (for example, a seat belt pressing on the prosthesis) may raise the possibility of prosthesis rupture. Certainly, if there has been a change in the way the breast feels or looks after trauma, then the possibility of rupture should be entertained.

WHAT TO DO IF YOUR PROSTHESIS HAS BEEN FOUND TO RUPTURE

The advice these days is that for whatever reason an investigation has been undertaken which reveals that your prosthesis has ruptured but you are happy with the present position in terms of size and how the breast feels, then really there is no indication to change the prosthesis. We now know that silicone is safe and your body will have made a scar – the capsule – around the prosthesis, which will contain the silicone (particularly if you have had cohesive gel implants inserted).

Across the globe, there are many thousands of women walking around who have had silicone breast prosthesis inserted that are leaking or have ruptured. There is no scientific evidence of risk to their wellbeing. Emotionally, however it is easy to understand that if something has broken inside your body you want to have it removed and a new prosthesis inserted.

Hardening of the breast and capsule formation

Until recent use of the ABBA Technique, cohesive gel implants or polyurethane implants there was a high incidence of capsular contracture (usually estimated to be one in ten patients) that will have sufficient hardening to spoil the result. We now know that this figure requires the duration of implantation to be considered because the longer the time, the increased chances of capsular contracture. All patients will have a degree of capsule formation because they all have a scar around the prosthesis; it is only when the capsule is hard and distorts the breast, or produces pain or an unpleasant feel to the breast that the patient demands treatment.

Treatment can be difficult and there are various options, as follows.

CLOSED CAPSULOTOMY

In days of old, closed capsulotomy was popular and involved squeezing the breast hard in the hope of breaking the contracted scar capsule. Unsurprisingly, there was a high incidence of rupturing the prosthesis too, especially when inserted under the muscle. There are a few cases of surgeons damaging their thumbs as well and so closed capsulotomy is no longer performed.

OPEN CAPSULOTOMY

This is the simplest surgical procedure and means the incision through which the prosthesis was inserted is opened and the scar capsule that your body has formed around the prosthesis is cut to allow the pocket to expand. This will result in the prosthesis and your breast initially feeling soft. However, the contracture in at least 50 per cent of cases will recur, meaning your breast will return to its hard state.

CAPSULECTOMY

If the capsule is thick, and this can only be decided at the time your breast has been opened at surgery, it may require complete removal. A capsulectomy may be complete or the anterior half only – 'anterior capsulectomy' – usually when submuscular as the posterior layer of capsule is firmly adherent to the ribs and intercostal muscles. This layer is very difficult to remove completely and risks both extra bleeding and possible damage to the intercostal muscles.

NEO-PLANE

A recent addition to the surgical possibilities has been the 'neo-plane', in which the capsule is dissected from the posterior surface of the breast but not removed. Why is this done? Capsulectomy is a difficult operation, which usually results in some of the breast tissue being removed, along with the capsule so an already small breast becomes even smaller. There is also far more bleeding associated with capsulectomy and we now know that the body converts blood in the pocket to fibrous scar tissue so further capsular contracture is more common. The neo-plane allows a fresh surface for the prosthesis and a reduction in the complications.

SALVAGE SURGERY

If there is breast droop, as well as capsular contracture

this is known as 'a rock in a sock' because it looks and feels just like a rock in a sock! As a consequence of the droop, a mastopexy procedure will also be required, thus surgical correction involves:

• Removal of prosthesis
• Capsulectomy or neo-plane dissection
• Reaugmentation
• Mastopexy

This is an involved procedure that takes several hours to undertake, has correspondingly higher rates of complication and is the most challenging area of breast augmentation surgery.

At the same time as any of the above surgical interventions, it is probably advisable for new implants to be inserted because infectious bacteria have been found in the biofilm (bacterial colony that exists on the surface of the implant) around implants that may cause later infection or recurrent capsular contracture. At this stage we tend to insert polyurethane-coated implants because the evidence is they have the lowest incidence of recurrent capsule formation.

Late swelling of the breast

Very occasionally after many years of successful breast augmentation, one or both breasts may suddenly swell for no apparent reason. This may result from:

• Infection elsewhere in the body, including flu

- Local low-grade infection from bacteria in the capsule, possibly coming through the nipple
- Spontaneous bleeding from the capsule not always caused by trauma
- Implant failure.

You should see your surgeon if this happens.

SCREENING

When it comes to screening, exactly the same guidelines apply for patients who have had breast augmentation as for the rest of the normal female population. It is dependent on family history, previous history of breast cancer and age.

Screening involves screening the implant and screening of the breast tissue. The implant is best screened with ultrasound and the breast tissue by a mammogram. Some patients complain about breast screening, particularly due to the fact that their breast has to be squeezed and they fear their breast prosthesis will be ruptured. Whilst we have yet to see a case proven that a prosthesis has been ruptured at the time of a mammogram it would not be inconceivable.

At your breast screening you should advise the radiographer that you have had a breast augmentation. Depending on the volume of the prosthesis and the size of your breasts, the silicone in the implants will cast a shadow. This can be overcome by doing different views.

It may be that your particular screening unit is inexperienced and will advise you to go along to another centre, where they are more likely to have previously screened patients with breast implants.

THE BOTTOM LINE

It is important that you remain under routine surveillance as for every other normal woman.

14
THE PATIENT'S PERSPECTIVE

NATASHA MOORE'S STORY
My personal motivation

As much as I love my two beautiful daughters and breastfed them both until they were nine months old, unfortunately this has taken its toll and my once pert, shapely breasts are empty and flatter than they used to be. I also yearn for a more hourglass figure as I am quite a small frame and have a tiny waist with a nice pair of hips, and I would love these to be in proportion with the rest of my body.

I'm a personal trainer and so I spend long hours in gymwear. To be more confident and proportionate in Lycra would be a great feeling and the thought of not having to boost my small boobs into uncomfortable plunge bras that feel like a corset, hurt like hell and dig into and mark my ribs would be utter bliss!

Feelings before the consultation

Having done a vast amount of research through the internet, talking to friends and friends of friends about different shapes, sizes, procedures and even how they felt, I knew the questions I personally wanted to ask beforehand so that I would be prepared for the consultation.

I was nervous and apprehensive revealing my boobs and having them examined and touched by a man I had never met before. It was somewhat bizarre – the only man to have done this for the past twelve years was my ex-husband!

The Cosmetic Surgery Partners Breast Clinic

Arriving at the clinic I was nervous and anxious but also strangely excited by the prospect of the end result. As the receptionist asked me to take a seat a million thoughts ran through my mind, especially what the surgeon would be like.

A very friendly nurse greeted me. She asked if this was my first time at the hospital (which it was) and I replied 'yes'. She then told me a little about the hospital and my surgeon, assuring me that I was in very capable hands (excuse the pun!).

Meeting my surgeon

I was greeted with a warm smile and a professional handshake. Although I was not sure what/who to expect, he was reassuring and made me feel at ease so much more than I could have expected – a completely professional gentleman with a sense of humour that eased the tension and anxiety I felt earlier.

We went through all my medical history in detail and completed the relevant forms. He took me through absolutely everything that I needed to know in a language I understood, from the possible side effects of the operation to explaining in detail, showing me the implants, and with a silk handkerchief surrounding the implant was able to demonstrate how scar tissue (the 'capsule') forms – very clever!

We talked at length and my questions were answered, including full explanation of the ABBA Technique used to minimise capsular contracture. I felt totally confident and informed about every aspect of the operation; I was delighted that I was to be treated by an excellent, experienced surgeon.

By this time I was comfortable and at ease in the surgeon's company so when asked to remove my top and bra for an examination and measurements, it felt less daunting. After several minutes with the ruler, great news – I have symmetrical boobs!

Trying the different-sized implants

Currently a 32B, I tried on a 32C bra – the sort of size I thought I might like to be. We started with small implants and this didn't make much of a difference; it just looked as though I was wearing a padded bra. Trying the different shapes was interesting, as I'd assumed the teardrop implant would provide a more natural shape for me. Then the round implants were brought out and after comparing the two, I was so much happier with the suggestion for these as they gave me the fuller and natural look I had dreamt of. Implants 330cc in volume were absolutely perfect and the exact shape and size I would love. I put my top on over the bra/implants and was so excited! They looked totally natural for my body shape.

As I looked at myself in the mirror I now saw a sexy, curvy hourglass and feminine shape. This is what the perfect pair looks like, I thought to myself. I looked at them from every possible angle in the mirror with the biggest smile. I did try some larger implants, but they were too large for me and personally not the natural look I was after as I did not want to have huge boobs or draw unnecessary attention. This helped confirm that I had made the correct choice in size.

Now overwhelmed by how well my consultation has gone with the most perfect boobs and excellent surgeon, I'm over the moon and make my next appointment for three weeks' time. Having left hospital I can hardly wait to tell my mum and close friends about the experience. I am bursting with excitement, as well as wanting to reassure them that I have every confidence in my decision to go ahead.

Now obsessed with boobs!

Since my decision to have the operation I have become so much more aware of other women's breasts. Just yesterday I asked a friend how she had such lovely boobs after having three children. I explained why I was asking her such a personal question; she went on to tell me the story of her boob job and how it has changed her life.

One friend told me how she no longer sleeps on her front and another couple of friends told me that they were initially shocked at the size and wondered, 'What have I done?' However, after a few weeks the swelling subsides and the final results are well worth it. I am glad that I am aware and prepared for the swelling; I have taken a lot from their experiences.

3D Imaging

I was completely unsure of what to expect when I arrived for 3D imaging and the machine looked more like a 6ft robot! The 3D machine took photos of my frame and dimensions of my body, taken at three different angles.

Once the photos were taken and shown back to me, I

was amazed – never before had I seen my body and boobs from such different angles! Being used to looking either straight down at my breasts or in a mirror, the 3D was able to project my boobs and body from so many different angles and from the angles that someone else would see me (men – wow!), it was incredible.

The 3D imaging gave me the opportunity to look and examine at length to allow me to come to the conclusion that my breasts were not currently in proportion with my otherwise curvy size 8 body.

Next, the 330cc implants were morphed onto my own body profile, showing me results from every angle. It took my breath away and verified that I had indeed made the perfect choice – they were everything I had imagined.

This procedure is fantastic and I would recommend any woman thinking of a boob job to try it and take a friend or partner with you for feedback. Could I be any more excited than I was already?! I am now totally confident and the 3D confirmed I was making the right decision for me.

The night before the operation

Wow, a huge mixture of emotions and feelings, mostly excitement that the big day is round the corner and happening at last! I feel very fortunate to have had such a positive experience in dealing with all staff at Simply Better Breasts.

Surprisingly I am not worried about the actual operation itself as I am happy that I've chosen the best surgeon for me. I have never had an operation before and am certainly not keen on needles, so am slightly apprehensive about the anaesthetic.

So, last drink for the evening before my early morning start and operation – so excited I can't sleep! I'm staying with a close friend and thinking of silly stuff, like if I should name my new boobs. Observing them in the mirror, saying this time tomorrow I am going to be even more of a woman than ever! Brings back awful memories of when I was a late developer at school and being teased and called names for having hardly any boobs.

The big day has finally arrived

Woke up early, bleary-eyed, as I really couldn't sleep last night. Quick shower and not amused at the prospect of wearing no make-up! Can't believe the day has arrived and I am so calm. So much so that I offer to drive us to London, singing all the way with my friend, who asks how I'm feeling – even she can't believe how relaxed I am. Arrive at the hospital happy to know that the lovely nurse will be looking after me today.

After filling in the forms unfortunately I have no option but to wear the awful-looking backless gown, paper knickers and tight knee-high socks. Definitely the most unglamorous look ever!

My surgeon arrives to go over the procedure, signs the consent form and makes the final markings on my chest, joking that I do indeed have no option but to wear the unattractive theatre outfit. I then meet the anaesthetist and am soon walking down to theatre and feeling surprisingly calm. In the theatre the radio is playing and the staff are really friendly. I lay down on the bed and my anaesthetist starts chatting away as if normal and I realise the needle has been put in almost without me noticing. He has a kind, soothing voice and tells me I will soon feel drowsy. And that is the last thing I remember...

Waking up after surgery

I remember the familiar voices of my surgeon and friend and ask, 'Have you done it yet?' as I can't feel any pain. Looking down, I see my bra in place and realise the operation is complete.

From what other women have told me about their experiences I expect to be in real pain and discomfort. I feel fine – no pain, relaxed, very tired (probably due to only a few hours' sleep the night before). I sleep upright on/off for a few hours. The nurse checked a few times to ensure I was comfortable and gave me some painkillers. My friends had said they were sick after the operation due to the anaesthetic and the antibiotics and painkillers made them poorly too, so I guess I was expecting that. I could not believe that within four hours of my operation

I was sat up in bed eating sandwiches, drinking coffee, and ice cream for dessert! I needed a little help to get my top back on as it was sore, lifting my arms up but other than that I felt much better than anticipated and headed home, driven by my friend. I took it easy for the rest of the day, propped up like the Queen of Sheba at my friend's house, and slept very well.

Day two

Woke up and now trying to get used to my new boobs. They are a combination of tight and heavy, and get in my way. Not in any pain, but they are swollen and seem so much bigger than what I am used to. My mum came to see me at my friend's house and could not believe how well I looked and would not have known I had had an operation the day before, other than the increased size.

I have a bath up to my waist, freshen up and head back home with my mum. Just twenty-four hours after the operation, Mum and I go for a celebratory dinner (small glass of wine, of course) and watch the sun set over the river. We cannot get over the fact that I feel so well.

Day three

Woke up and my boobs have swollen a little bit more. If I had not spoken to people beforehand I would be worried that they look so large but I know it's very early days and this will settle. Also, I think the bras I bought were probably not the best. Sport-support bras that go over the head, doing up at the back are far more difficult than front-fasteners and this is the one thing I would like to have known preoperatively.

I needed to go shopping for some more suitable clothes and underwear for the warm summer weather and not sure why but felt very emotional today, to the point that I am in a shop and start to cry, which is very unlike me. Think it may be a mixture of missing my daughters while they are away and not having my usual exercise as an outlet. My mum and I decide to enjoy another dinner out and an early night.

Day four

Today the bra I am wearing is much more comfortable. The dress I am wearing also fits me so much better than it used to, although it is still a size 8. My new boobs change my figure and clothes so much, my dress looks much more alluring than ever before. I have worn this dress often, but I felt so different in it today. My new shape makes me feel more confident and my clothes seem to fit as they should have done with all the curves in the right places!

Walking down the street a group of guys stop and look at me, one asking, 'Will you marry me?' Not sure whether it is a coincidence but never have I had a proposal on the street before and I feel quite flattered.

THE PATIENT'S PERSPECTIVE

Day five
The support strap has been a bit itchy for the past few days, with the weather being so warm, and I'm getting hot and sweaty, which means it is peeling off. I think the painkillers have made me constipated so am very happy when, having phoned the nurse, I am able to remove the support band with care and discontinue the painkillers.

Day seven
I have not told my daughters about my operation as I worry that they are too young to understand. They have been at their grandparents for the week – really missed them terribly. Missing my job as a personal trainer and feeling quite frustrated at not being able to exercise but then I look down at my new boobs and know that they are more than worth a month's sacrifice.

I have found that I have a greater sense of confidence throughout this whole experience and not just with my appearance, if that makes sense.

Day eight: hospital check-up
I put on a dress again today as it was hot and it used to look nice on me before. Now it looks amazing and not having to wear a padded bra ever again is such an amazing feeling! I meet the nurse and mention that my left boob is slightly higher, larger and harder than the right, which is softer, less swollen and has dropped slightly. She tells me that it is nothing to worry about

– it's just that the swelling on the left is taking longer to go down than the right and this is normal.

She also gives me a few hints about bras (best type and where to get them), deodorants (roll-on, not spray), shower-gel (not too perfumed) and after a month to massage the scars.

I leave content and am looking forward to the swelling going down and them dropping slightly – then I will be ecstatic!!

Week two

I drove to Wales on day nine and my boobs felt tight, very firm and numb, which has taken me a while to get used to. It's a strange feeling and at the moment I have no sensation in my nipples.

Aware of the long drive and a tight seat belt across my chest, I drove for three hours with a cushion under the seat belt and had no problems.

I met up with some friends for the evening and wore a dress that is high-necked but fits in all the right places. Their comments were all positive as they know the size I was before and think the new breasts really suit me. Also, they agree that I have chosen the right size for the natural look as if they had never met me before, they would think I had amazing boobs and not think I'd had a boob job.

My family's reactions were also very positive, with my mum, sister, aunty and even my grandmother requesting a viewing! All were surprised that although swollen they still look like my boobs, just slightly bigger and much fuller. They said that they were expecting a stuck-on Victoria Beckham kind of look, however they thought mine looked far more natural than anything they have seen in magazines, etc.

Week two, and I spoke to my surgeon by telephone as the left remains slightly higher, firmer and larger. Fortunately, he assured me that this is completely normal and by week six they should have settled. Still no feeling in my nipples yet but apparently this is normal at first, too.

Week three

I am really getting to know and feel at ease with my boobs. I am now able to sleep for periods of time on my sides. At last I have my nipples back! They are feeling the cold and reacting exactly as they should. The skin is no longer numb and they are definitely feeling softer and more like my own. Looking in the mirror I feel so lucky – I still can't believe they are mine to keep! In everything I wear, I feel delighted with my new figure.

Cannot describe how pleased I am to have done this; the whole experience has been interesting, liberating and an amazing journey that will continue. The people who have been on this journey with me, from my closest friend to my surgeon, can all see not just the amazing results of my now-perfect pair but also the big smile and confidence that come with it. Looking forward to no longer wearing the support bras and going on a spree for a sultry new underwear collection, new bikinis and the kind of clothes that would now look amazing with my shape, including backless and strapless dresses. The list is endless and very exciting!!!

Weeks six to eight

My boobs are now a part of me and I think and feel differently about them. They have dropped and softened and look amazing, perfect and natural. Having shown a few of my friends, all responses have been impressive and they can't believe how natural they look – from where they are standing, they can't even see the scars. Initially (first few weeks), they didn't feel or look real and they didn't quite seem my own. Now, however, they feel and look natural and are now in my mind absolutely and completely a part of me.

As all women should, I love shopping for clothes and underwear, and now it's even more enjoyable than ever before! My underwear collection used to consist of uncomfortable, padded bras, but now I have bought lots of new underwear and pretty lace bras are a favourite. So much more confident and happy with my body, this is the best it's ever looked!

My first 'bedroom' experience with my new boobs felt very different for me. Whereas before being naked for the first time with someone (although I feel happy with my body), I was not overly confident about my boobs. Well, this has totally changed and I feel so much more confident about my body than ever before. The response was everything I had hoped for, and more.

I now fill blouses in all the right places and one dress I bought is just stunning. I love it so much – it's figure hugging, classy but very sexy, and I can honestly say I have never felt so good in a dress. Wearing dresses with no bra at all for the first time in ten years is liberating and an amazing feeling!

Three months on

I'm feeling on top of the world with life and my absolutely perfect pair! They've fulfilled all my high expectations. I find myself looking in the mirror, staring – still can't believe how perfect they are and that they are mine to keep forever. I feel incredibly lucky and overjoyed with my overall figure, experience and the whole journey. Now three months on, my amazing boobs are really soft to touch. They look so much more natural than the early days and truly a part of me now. No one would know! This is exactly the result I dreamt of.

15

BRAS AND BEYOND

A brassière, or bra for short, is an article of clothing that covers, supports and elevates the breasts. Bras are worn for cultural, comfort and, at times, concealment reasons. Originally purely functional, they are now more fashion-orientated and have both erotic and symbolic significance. The industry has grown and makes billions of pounds annually. Manufacturers play on the importance that many Western women place on body image, particularly their breast shape.

The functions of the brassière are numerous:
• Coverage
• Support and elevation
• Shape improvement

- Change in size and shape perception (larger or smaller)
- Restraint during exercise
- To produce or enhance cleavage
- Assist with nursing
- Eroticism
- Symbolic of 'coming of age'
- Political, i.e. 'bra-burning'.

A BRIEF HISTORY

The origin of the word 'brassière' is actually ancient French from when an 'arm protector' (*bracière* – bras being French for 'arm') came to encompass a breastplate as part of a suit of armour and subsequently a female corset. Interestingly, while the English-speaking world has kept the term, usually abbreviated to bra, the French currently know it as a *soutien-gorge* – literally, a throat support. Mind you, this is coming from the nation that refers to flat, droopy breasts as *gants de toilette* – toilet gloves!

Recorded history of the use of something as coverage or protection for the female breast extends as far back as female athletes in the 14th century BC Minoan era. China's Ming Dynasty used cloth with cups and shoulder straps tied to a belt around the back – the 'doudou'. The most common female undergarment, especially of the wealthier class, from the 1500s was the corset, due to its ability to elevate the breasts in addition to shaping the waist.

The first of what we would recognise as today's brassières appeared in the early 20th century. This signalled the end of the corset and the start of the multi-billion-pound bra industry. Styles have, of course, changed according to the prevailing fashions of the day. The 1920s saw the 'Flapper' era, where breasts were flattened and concealed as much as possible. Jane Russell's 'bullet' bra worn in *The Outlaw* (1943) is fairly self-explanatory and no doubt provided the inspiration for Jean Paul Gaultier's famous conical bra, sported by Madonna in the 1990s.

It is said that the bra celebrated its centenary in 2010, first appearing in *Vogue* magazine in 1907, and was formalised by inclusion into 1911's *Oxford English Dictionary*. There is some confusion, but it would appear that the first bra to be patented (1914) was attributed to Mary Phelps Jacobs, a New York socialite who also used the business nom de plume 'Caresse Crosby'. Disliking the constrictive corsets du jour, her invention comprised a pair of handkerchiefs (naturally, silk), tied together in the middle and with silk ribbons stitched on as shoulder straps. Although her fellow females did not share her enthusiasm at the time, Warners turned the reported purchase price of $1,500 into more than $15m over the next thirty years.

1893   The appearance of the term 'brassière' in the English language

1904   First use of the term by manufacturers
1907   First use by *Vogue* magazine
1911   Included in *The Oxford English Dictionary*
1914   Initial patent by Mary Phelps Jacob
1930   Shortened to 'bra'
1960s Padding and underwiring added
1994   The 'Wonderbra' is introduced
2001   A metal-free 'frequent-flyer' bra is introduced

STRUCTURE

A brassière comprises numerous constituent parts, including:

- Two cups
- One gore (the central panel connecting the cups)
- One band
- Two shoulder straps

The bra marked a seismic shift in approach: whereas corsets flattened or pushed up the bust from below, the bra aims to support the breasts from above. In fact, the latest designs may combine the two to maximise cleavage and gives rise to the slang term 'cleavage caddies'.

One thing that males completely fail to understand is the concept of an 'underwire bra'. This is a curved piece of metal (or plastic) that provides additional support for the cups and frequently blocks the washing machine drain, if not removed prior to washing.

Another thing that often catches the male of the

species unawares is the 'Wonderbra' that enhances the cleavage, either by cantilevering or additional padding. Made famous by Eva Herzigova's traffic-stopping 'Hello Boys' advertising campaign of 1997, it has led the occasional man to 'wonder' where the breasts disappeared to after removal of the bra!

DESIGN

If 'structure' implies some sort of mechanical engineering, then it is not too far away as bra designers share with bridge-designers the need to work with similar forces: indeed, bras have been likened to suspension bridges. Both suffer strongly from gravitational forces – i.e. pulling down towards the ground – but also torsional and tangential forces produced when the wearer turns or twists. Correctly fitted, the band and underwire should do the majority of the work. If incorrect, the shoulders will bear the brunt of the weight, particularly with large breasts, and produce neck, back and shoulder pain in later life.

Calculating volume

The breast being a three-dimensional structure, manufacturers have used a variety of methods of calculating volume in order to create bras, but all rely on some elementary mathematics. Bra designers can calculate the volume of a brassière cup in several ways, depending on the shape of the breast. If the breast is round and essentially the shape of a half-sphere, any of three formulae might be used:

$$V = \frac{2\pi r^3}{3} \text{ so } V = 2.1 \times r^3 \text{ or } V = 0.26 \times D^3$$

Where V equals the volume of one-half sphere, D equals the diameter of the sphere, and r equals the radius of the sphere.

If the breast is shaped more like a cone, the designer might use a formula such as the following:

$$V = 0.26 \times D_b^2 \times h$$

Where Db equals the diameter of the cone's base and h equals the height of the cone. [Display ends]

Other formulae can be derived as needed to design bras for differently shaped breasts.

The defining characteristic of a bra is its ability to lift the breast from its normal position of lying on the lower chest/upper abdominal wall and to keep it there. Far from being simply pairs of cups and straps connected by a band, the modern bra is more of a high-tech engineering solution than a protector of female modesty. Commonly used fabrics include cotton, polyester, Spandex and lace although other, cooler alternatives have been tried.

Fastening is generally through hooks and eyes, plastic clasps or occasionally, Velcro, and is uncommon at the front. This rear-fastening neatly divides females into the 'spinners' (those who fasten the bra at the front, then shuffle it round to the back) and the 'contortionists' (those who manage it blind behind their backs). Most men are usually baffled by both techniques, but then it might be fair to say their attention could be elsewhere.

Think of the image of a suspension bridge and you will easily comprehend why bra designers use similar principles to cantilevered-bridge construction: both are affected in the vertical dimension by gravitational forces. Horizontal forces – wind and earth movement in a bridge, twisting and bending the torso in the bra – must also be taken into account. The 1964 treatise entitled 'Brassières: an engineering miracle' of one Edward Nanas exhibited quasi-reverential enthusiasm: 'in supporting a semi-solid, variable volume mass in addition to its adjacent mirror image, the female bosom involves a design effort comparable to a cantilevered skyscraper. As any large-breasted woman knows well, it is important to have a well-engineered and well-fitting bra otherwise the shoulders take an excess share of the workload, precipitating back pain with time as the erstwhile supporting structure behaves as a pulley.'

Fitting

With studies estimating 80 per cent of British women to

have incorrectly fitting bras, it may be useful to summarise the key features of the optimally fitted bra:

- The band should always be horizontal and firm but not uncomfortably so. A common error is to have it riding up at the back rather than being parallel to the floor.
- Note: the band forms the primary support to the breasts and is very important. The underwire of each cup should lay flat on the chest wall, *not* the breast. It should lie exactly in the inframammary fold (IMF) without poking inwards or protruding outwards.
- The breast mounds should be comfortably contained by the cups, the fabric forming a smooth line with the upper pole of the breast. Neither should bulge out of the top (indicating the bra is too small) nor allow the cup to collapse inwards (the cup is too large).
- The centre of the cup should house the nipple; the apex of the breast shoulder straps should neither cut in nor slip off and are not primarily designed to support the weight of the breast, 80 per cent of which should be provided by the band and cups. It should allow comfortable breathing and easy movement without slippage.

THE RIGHT BRA

As every woman knows, finding the correct bra does seem to be a challenge, with many chains and stores appearing to have completely different reference points. Also, the female breast is almost infinitely variable in size, shape, volume and contour.

The two key measurements are:

- Band – taken horizontally around the chest, just beneath the breast. Many fail to comprehend that this number has little or nothing to do with the breast but everything to do with the underlying chest wall. This is a linear measurement so those who at consultation confidently request a 32X or 36Y have not quite grasped the concept.
- Cup size – also measured around the chest, but this time including the breast at its most protuberant part, i.e. the nipple. Unlike the band, this is not linear but a 3D, volumetric assessment is an indicator of the breast's voluptuousness. It is the most important, but most difficult part of evaluation.

The system for sizing then requires some mental gymnastics so it is not at all surprising that bra-wearers are confused. Indeed, one method of measurement requires the wearer to start by wearing a perfectly fitting bra! A study in the *British Journal of Plastic Surgery* from 2003 found that the most common error was too large a cup (on average, three sizes) and too small a band (on average, four) in a series of women awaiting breast reduction surgery.

While accurate fitting is the area of greatest difficulty, it is not necessarily always a feature of poor design but the sheer breadth of variability in individual breasts, their size, shape, volume, distribution and position on a chest wall, which has its own particular characteristics. Imagine trying to build a straight house on an uneven piece of ground! Moreover, a similar volume of breast may have a widely varying cup-size classification.

A further confounding feature is the symmetry – that is, the degree by which a person's breasts are identical, or otherwise. In fact, surgeons have long appreciated that some degree of difference between a woman's two breasts is, in fact, the norm. An American study indicated that some degree of observable asymmetry occurred in up to 80 per cent of women. Although many women volunteer a difference during consultation, others remain completely unaware until a surgeon points out sometimes quite obvious differences.

As anyone who has trudged the length of Oxford Street will attest, it is more than a little frustrating that manufacturers seem unable to agree on a standard brassière scale. Moreover, some artificially inflate their sizes in a subtle psychological inducement to sales. On the other hand, the infinite variability of female breasts means that manufacturers can only really produce a range of standard sizes that are a 'close fit' rather than exact.

Bras have also been used to make a political statement: the classic 'bra-burning' of Germaine Greer's feminist movement at the vanguard against the misogynist male of the 1960s. This is curious in a garment first designed by a woman. In fact, half the patents filed for bra designs have been from women themselves.

16

FURTHER INFORMATION AND USEFUL CONTACTS

BREAST AUGMENTATION (BA): FAQS

Q. How long does the operation take?
A. Although some surgeons aim for minutes, a good-quality BA takes up to one hour.

Q. Can it be done under local anaesthetic?
A. Technically, yes, but for reasons of comfort and safety a brief general anaesthetic is preferred.

Q. Can it be done as a day case?
A. Yes, it is very common to have BA as a day case, but it is wise not to travel too far from the hospital on the first night in the rare event of a complication.

Q. Will I have wound drains?

A. No, it is neither necessary nor preferred with respect to encapsulation rates to have drains for a primary BA. It is, however, usual to have drains – usually for only twenty-four hours – when secondary or revision surgery has been performed.

Q. Will it hurt?

A. That depends on many factors, including the individual's pain threshold and the technique employed, but today's best procedures usually give little or no pain. The vast majority of women are able to return to their activities of daily living the very next day.

Q. Is it more painful under the muscle?

A. Again, if done properly there is no reason why it should be more painful, although there are some patients who have intertwined muscles that may be more sore for a day or so afterwards.

Q. What is the recovery time?

A. One should be back to normal activities within a day or two, but driving should be left for a week and aerobic exercise or the gym four to six weeks. You should be back at work after a week, but this may be influenced by exactly what job you do.

Q. Are there any complications?
A. As it is a surgical procedure there is the potential for unwanted consequences such as bleeding and infection, which are rare. Your surgeon should discuss these in detail with you before surgery.

Q. What is 'hardening' and is it dangerous?
A. Also known as 'rejection', 'encapsulation' and 'adverse capsular contracture', this is simply the body's response to any implant (such as heart valves, neurological shunts and the like), whereby protective scar tissue seals off the foreign body. In a small minority (between 2 and 5 per cent), this natural reaction will be more active and cause the breast to appear firm. While not dangerous, it can distort the breast and affect the cosmetic result.

Q. How will I scar, where will it be and can I help it in any way?
A. How each individual scars depends on many factors, including genetics. Look at any other scars you have, either from surgery or trauma, to give yourself an idea. The most common site nowadays is in the crease beneath the breast, but some prefer the armpit. The only thing that we know helps to speed scar maturation is massage.

Q. How long will the prosthesis last?
A. Today's implants are fifth generation and the result of nearly fifty years' continual development. Scientific studies indicate that they are much more durable than their predecessors, but no exact figures are available. We have stopped recommending replacement every ten years.

Q. Will I require surgery in the future?
A. That depends on many factors but remember the breast is an active organ that changes not only with age, but each month with hormonal cycles and with pregnancy and breastfeeding. As the prostheses continually improve in quality and durability, implant rupture becomes less frequent so an altered breast around the implant will be more common.

Q. Am I a suitable candidate?
A. If medically fit, with no health problems, there should be no particular reason why not but each patient should be individually assessed. Each patient should be well enough informed to balance the risks and benefits of any surgical procedure.

Q. Will the final result be visible straight after the operation?
A. It is important to understand that each patient will react differently and a teenager with small breasts will

be very different to a mature mother who has had several children and breastfed them. They often appear too high and too round in the first few weeks, but settle over three to six months as the tissues adjust to the new weight and volume.

Q. Why should I take the prescribed antibiotics?
A. While important to fight against infection (which usually causes loss of the implant), the latest research indicates that antibiotics both during and after surgery can reduce the frequency of capsular hardening.

Q. How can I check the surgeon's experience?
A. There are several things that can be checked, but all surgeons in the UK must be on the GMC register, ideally the Specialist Register for Plastic Surgery. Those trained in the UK will have the FRCS (Plast), a fellowship of the Royal College of Surgeons with specialist training in plastic and reconstructive surgery. The surgeon should be undertaking such surgery on a regular basis and be able to show a range of results, good and not so good, from previous patients.

ANAESTHESIA: FAQS

Q. I am frightened of having an anaesthetic – how dangerous is it?
A. General anaesthesia is extremely safe for fit and

healthy patients. You will be carefully assessed to ensure you have no health problems that would increase your anaesthetic risk. Anaesthetists are doctors who have undergone specialist training in anaesthesia and are very experienced in anaesthesia for cosmetic surgery.

Q. Why do I need to stop eating and drinking before the operation?
A. You are starved to reduce the risk of you being sick during the operation and then breathing it into your lungs. It is vital that you do not eat for six hours prior to surgery. Pre-op, water can be drunk up to two hours when taking tablets. This applies to general anaesthesia and sedation.

Q. Can I have a local anaesthetic?
A. Some minor procedures may be done under local anaesthetic. This can be discussed with your surgeon at the consultation stage.

Q. I'd like to be asleep, but not have a full general anaesthetic – what about sedation?
A. Sedation means different things to different people. Light sedation can make you more comfortable and reduce anxiety during surgery under local anaesthesia. You will be able to talk and obey instructions throughout the procedure but you will also be sleepy.

Often people have reduced memory of the surgery. Deep sedation when you are fully asleep is really anaesthesia and uses the same drugs. There is no evidence that it is safer or better. Your anaesthetist will be happy to discuss your options by telephone prior to your admission.

Q. Will I need lots of investigations?
A. Usually, fit and healthy people below the age of sixty do not require any tests. If you are over sixty or have other health problems, some simple tests will be required. Please bring copies of any letters and test results you have from your GP or specialist so that we can avoid unnecessarily repeating tests.

Q. I'm afraid of dying during the operation.
A. Death under anaesthesia is very, very rare but this is a frequent fear. We all have risks in our daily lives that we accept and rarely think about, e.g. car or air travel. Anaesthesia is extremely safe. During the anaesthetic your anaesthetist will be watching your heartbeat, blood pressure, oxygen level and breathing the whole time. He/she is with you and looking after you all the time.

Q. Will I wake up during the operation?
A. The level of anaesthesia is constantly monitored when you are asleep and adjusted to ensure you are not

receiving too much or too little. Awareness can occur but is very rare for this type of anaesthetic.

Q. Will I have a pre-med?
A. No. Premeds are not normally used in modern anaesthetic practice, which most people prefer. If you are especially nervous and want a premed, please discuss this prior to admission.

Q. I have had anaesthetics before but I feel particularly anxious about this one. Can you help?
A. Having a cosmetic operation is not the same as having your appendix out! It is your choice and not necessary for your health. This makes most people much more worried about the anaesthetic, so really you are normal. We understand how stressed you can feel and will do our best to support you. Your safety and wellbeing are very important to us and you can be assured of the highest level of care.

Q. I am a needle phobic – will I have to have any injections?
A. No one likes needles! If you are afraid of pain you can have a local anaesthetic cream, which makes it pain-free. Please request this early as it takes about forty-five minutes to be fully effective. Intravenous anaesthesia is safer and smoother so we do not recommend going to sleep with gas.

Q. But I have difficult veins...

A. Your anaesthetist is very experienced, skilled and an expert in difficult veins.

Q. I don't like masks...

A. You may be asked to breathe oxygen before you go to sleep but you do not have to have it by a facemask. Oxygen is very important and is given routinely when you wake up. Again, you do not have to have it by mask.

Q. I smoke, is this a problem?

A. Smoking, especially more than five cigarettes a day can increase the risk of anaesthetic complications. You will be advised to stop all smoking before your operation, ideally for six weeks. This will significantly reduce the risk of chest infection. If this is not possible, it is extremely important not to smoke for twenty-four hours pre-admission or for seventy-two hours post-operatively.

Q. I take regular medication prescribed by my doctor – should I continue taking it?

A. Please continue all regular medication as normal; this includes tablets and inhalers. The only exceptions are the antidepressants in the group called 'monoamine oxidase inhibitors'. These are rarely prescribed and you will have been given a card because you must avoid certain foods. Tablets can be taken with a small sip of water. It is important to have a full list of all medicines taken in the last six months.

Q. What about non-prescription medications, including herbal remedies and recreational drugs?

A. Please inform us of all medication. Some herbal remedies, e.g. St John's wort, can interact with other drugs and should be stopped. Recreational substances can be extremely dangerous with anaesthetics – especially cocaine, which should not be taken within seven days of your operation.

Q. I have asthma, is it a risk?

A. If your asthma is well controlled, this should not be a problem. Please continue with your inhalers and check your peak flow. If you feel wheezy or have a cold, your surgery may need to be postponed until you are well again.

Q. I am overweight, is this dangerous?

A. Being moderately overweight is not a contraindication to anaesthesia. However, if you have other problems such as diabetes or high blood pressure this can increase overall risk. Ideally, weight loss of a few kilos and some regular exercise, e.g. walking, can help, but we recognise this may be unrealistic. Deep vein thrombosis is rare but you will probably require some extra peri-operative anti-thrombosis treatment.

Cosmetic surgery is not life saving and so minimising risk is important.

Q. I am diabetic, what should I do?
A. This will depend on whether your condition is managed with insulin, tablets and/or diet. The key is being well-controlled. This will be discussed preoperative assessment and a management plan will be made.

Q. Can I have my operation as a day case?
A. Some procedures can be done as a day case. You will need to have a responsible adult to take you home and look after you for twenty-four hours post discharge. Postoperatively, you will need to stay a minimum of four hours. If you live more than sixty minutes away by car, it is recommended to stay overnight.

Q. Will I be sick?
A. We routinely give anti-sickness medication to prevent nausea and vomiting. It is never 100 per cent effective, so if you have suffered nausea and vomiting after anaesthetics please discuss it preoperatively so any adjustments can be made.

Q. Why am I asked if I have any caps, crowns, bridges, loose teeth or veneers?
A. Artificial teeth may not be as strong as natural teeth

so there is a small risk of dental damage. Your anaesthetist needs to know where these teeth are in your mouth so they can be protected, where possible.

Q. Will the operation be painful?
A. Many cosmetic procedures are relatively pain-free. You will receive painkillers while you are asleep, as well as some local anaesthetic. Painkillers will be prescribed for you after your operation and to take home.

Q. Are you experienced in this type of surgery?
A. Your anaesthetist and surgeon work together as a team, often for many years. All the anaesthetists are very experienced in this field. Your safety and wellbeing is our priority.

Q. When will I meet my anaesthetist?
A. You will meet the anaesthetist on the ward on the day of your operation. A full assessment will be made, which will involve answering questions you have already been asked. Please bear with us: we want to get to know you and form a full picture of you and your needs. You will meet us again in the anaesthetic room and again when you have woken up. We are available for postoperative advice.

Q. I would like to talk over the anaesthetic before I commit to the surgery or pre-admission. Is this possible?

FURTHER INFORMATION AND USEFUL CONTACTS

A. We are always happy to do telephone consultations. Please discuss this with your surgeon, who will arrange it. Sometimes it may be necessary to make an outpatient appointment.

Q. Do you have any other advice?

A. Please help us to help you! We need to be fully informed and request that you comply with any pre- or postoperative instructions. We aim to make your operation and recovery as safe as possible. If, in the extremely unlikely event you are cancelled on the day of surgery, this will be for your safety. It is a team effort, between your surgeon and anaesthetist, with you at the centre.

17

USEFUL CONTACTS

The Care Quality Commission (CQC)
St Nicholas Building
St Nicholas Street
Newcastle upon Tyne
NE1 1NB
Tel: 03000 616161
Email: enquiries@cqc.org.uk

The General Medical Council
3 Hardman Street
Manchester
M3 3AN
Website: www.gmc-uk.org (check online complaints).

Get in touch with Action Against Medical Accidents (AVMA) for further help, if you are dissatisfied with the service received for whatever reason: www.avma.org.uk (tel: 0845 123 2352). They will help you through their very informative website and pursue the appropriate channel.

Independent Healthcare Advisory Services (IHAS)
Centre Point
103 New Oxford Street
WC1A 1DU
Tel: 020 7379 8598
Email: info@independenthealthcare.org.uk

Simply Better Breasts
Follow us on Facebook at:
www.facebook.com/pages/Simply-Better-
Breasts/226291517397554 or on Twitter @sbbreasts

The Trading Standards Institute
1 Sylvan Court
Sylvan Way
Southfields Business Park
Basildon
Essex SS15 6TH
Tel: 0845 4040506
Website:
www.tradingstandards.gov.uk/advice/consumer-
advice.cfm or visit the Directgov website:
www.direct.gov.uk/en/Governmentcitizensandrights/Co
nsumerrights/index.htm

18

GLOSSARY

ABBA – American anti-Biotic Breast Augmentation

ACC – adverse capsular contracture

Aplasia (hypoplasia) – lack of development

Axilla/Axillary tail – armpit/projection of part of the breast into the armpit

Body Dysmorphic Disorder – a condition whereby the affected person has an excessive concern and preoccupation with a perceived defect of a physical features

Capsule – the fibrous 'bag' of scar tissue that forms around a breast implant

CTD – connective tissue disorder

Cooper's ligaments – supporting fibrous tissue structures of the breast

Dual-plane (aka biplanar) – a technique, originally

developed by John Tebbetts, that places the prosthesis beneath the muscle at the top and under the gland at the bottom. It may be used for mild-to-moderate degrees of ptosis

DVT – deep vein thrombosis

Elastomer – the outer shell of the implant

Gel bleed – leakage of the implant's filler gel

Haematoma – a collection of blood within a surgical pocket that, if sufficiently large and expanding, may require surgical removal

Hypertrophy – growth, usually excessive, for example in a scar

IMF – inframammary fold

Mastopexy – also known as an uplift

NAC – nipple-areola complex

Necrosis – tissue death, usually as a result of inadequate blood supply

Ptosis – droop or sag in response to gravity

Seroma – a collection of tissue fluid that may require surgical drainage

Symmastia – aka synmastia (also, uniboob, bread-loaf breast) is a confluence of the breasts so that the normal cleavage is obliterated

TIVA – Total Intra-Venous Anaesthesia

Tubular/tuberose – a congenital abnormality of the breast involving some degree of underdevelopment of the gland and enlargement or herniation of the NAC

GLOSSARY

ACRONYMS

BAAPS – British Association of Aesthetic Plastic Surgeons

BACD – British Association of Cosmetic Doctors

BAPRAS – British Association of Plastic, Reconstructive & Aesthetic Surgeons

BCAM – British College of Aesthetic Medicine

CQC (formerly HCC – Healthcare Commission) – Care Quality Commission

FDA – Food and Drug Administration: the American body responsible for drug and medical device regulation

GMC – General Medical Council

IHAS – Independent Health Advisory Service

IRG – Independent Review Group

ISAPS – International Society of Aesthetic Plastic Surgery

PCT – primary care trust

PIP – Poly Implant Prothèse

RCS (FRCS) – Royal College of Surgeons (Fellow RCS)

19

FURTHER READING

1. *Enhancing patient outcomes in aesthetic and reconstructive breast surgery using triple antibiotic breast irrigation: six-year prospective clinical study.* Adams WP, Rios JL, Smith SJ. *Plast Reconstr Surg* 2006; 117: 30-6
2. *Vertical scar breast reduction with medial flap or glandular transposition of the nipple-areola.* Asplund OA, Davies DM. *Br J Plast Surg* 1996; 49: 507-14
3. *Breast augmentation: part I – a review of the silicone prosthesis.* MG Berry, DM Davies. *J Plast Reconstr Aesth Surg* 2010; 63: 1761-68
4. *Breast augmentation: part II – adverse capsular contracture.* MG Berry, V Cucchiara, DM Davies. *J Plast Reconstr Aesth Surg* 2010; 63: 2098-107
5. *Breast augmentation: part III – preoperative*

considerations and planning. MG Berry, V Cucchiara, DM Davies. *J Plast Reconstr Aesth Surg* 2011; 64: 1401-1409

6. *The Ultimate Cleavage: a practical guide to cosmetic breast enlargement surgery.* Heasman MK. 1999 ISBN 0953542408

7. *An investigation of the suitability of bra fit in women referred for reduction mammaplasty.* Greenbaum AR, Heslop T, Morris J, Dunn KW. *Br J Plast Surg* 2003; 56: 230-6

8. *Breast augmentation with anatomical cohesive gel implants.* Hedén P, Jernbeck J, Hober M. *Clin Plast Surg* 2001; 28: 531-52

9. *Local complications after cosmetic breast implant surgery in Finland.* Kulmala I, McLaughlin JK, Pakkanen M, Lassila K, Hölmich LR, Lipworth L, Boice JD Jr, Raitanen J, Luoto R. Ann Plast Surg 2004; 53: 413-9

10. *Anatomical and artistic breast considerations.* Moufarrège R. *Ann Chir Plast Esthet* 2005; 50:365-70

11. *Partially submuscular breast augmentation.* Regnault P. *Plast Reconstr Surg* 1977; 59: 72-6

12. *Motivational factors and psychological processes in cosmetic breast augmentation surgery.* Solvi AS, Foss K, von Soest T, Roald HE, Skolleborg KC, Holte A. *J Plast Reconstr Aesthet Surg* 2010; 63: 673-80

13. *A system for breast implant selection based on patient tissue characteristics and implant-soft tissue*

dynamics. Tebbetts JB. *Plast Reconstr Surg* 2002; 109: 1410-5

14. *A history of the breast*. Yalom M. Ballantine Books, 1998

15. http://www.mhra.gov.uk/home/groups/dts-bi/ documents/websiteresources /con2032510.pdf

16. http://www.mhra.gov.uk/Safetyinformation/ Generalsafetyinformationandadvice/Product-specificinformationandadvice/Product-specificinformationandadvice-A-F/Breastimplants /index.htm